Praise for Malissa Keisch and
Life Tumbled

"Malissa is like the fun, warm, and responsible aunt every girl needs. Her book offers young women encouragement and practical tips in a conversational, relatable way."

—**Chelsea Johnson**, Licensed Independent Marriage and Family Therapist

"Whether you have helicopter parents who taught you everything or parents who have given you more space than you would like, you will want to read this book as you navigate the transition into adulthood. The advice is solid and up-to-date.

"In true Malissa form, this book presents direction with love and acceptance. I have known Malissa for almost ten years. She is one of the women I admire most both professionally and personally. She gives everything 200 percent and isn't afraid to be authentic. She is real, comforting, full of love, and ready to get her hands dirty. These traits allow her to excel in areas that many are too afraid to even attempt. Her commitment to excellence and loving herself and others for who they are is infectious. If you know Malissa, you want to be around her; to gleam a little of the magic she possesses and gives so freely of. As a Christian mother myself, I find her advice on point with how I want my own child raised. Thank you, Malissa, for this amazing guidebook."

—**Jessica Elgin**, Real Estate Agent

"*Life Tumbled* offers great insights to help others, specifically young women, discover their potential and individuality. It inspires the reader to seek within themselves and question the depth of their existence. Within the pages, the seeker will be provided with helpful tools, information, and questions to encourage their curiosity and take advantage of their life right now.

"The author's willingness to share vulnerable experiences allows for a relatable conversion to take place. Even though she belongs to one specific religion, Malissa is quick to include any young women in need of guidance and love; no matter what their background might be. *Life Tumbled* is written from a genuine perspective of love; and where there is love, there is God because God is love. No matter what season of life you are in, do not pass up this book; it is well worth you time."

—**Ashley Veater**, Student

"*Life Tumbled* is real, true, and relatable. Malissa's story is generous in its detail and transparent in its assessments of life. Malissa has bravely shared the triumphs and tribulations, the victories and the pain, all in equal measure. With an openness of spirit, she gives her journey to us so we don't have to learn the hard way."

—**Melissa Forziat**, Marketer, www.melissaforziatevents.com

"This book is truly a breath of fresh air filled with honest and real perspectives in life. It is a practical guide to an area of life that isn't often taught—the ability to transition from a teen to an adult. I cannot wait for so many others to have their minds opened and hearts softened as a result of reading these pages. I know of Malissa's character and integrity. In a world of many fake role models, she exemplifies *Life Tumbled* as a ray of light in having optimism through life's trials. This book is a healing perspective for all youth and parents alike. For me as a husband and father of four, Malissa is helping prepare my family and I for future events we will experience. I am truly inspired in reading *Life Tumbled* and excited to share this book with so many others!"

—**Dwain Schallenberger**, Real Estate Agent

Life
Tumbled

Life Tumbled

How Christian Young Women
Can Feel Confident, Find Love,
Make a Living, Grow Spiritually,
and Survive Life's Grit

MALISSA KELSCH

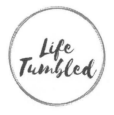

Life Tumbled LLC

St. George, UT

Life Tumbled LLC
St. George, UT
www.lifetumbled.com
Send feedback to malissa@lifetumbled.com

Publisher's Cataloging-In-Publication Data

    Names: Kelsch, Malissa, author.
    Title: Life tumbled : how Christian young women can feel confident, find love, make a living, grow spiritually, and survive life's grit / Malissa Kelsch.
    Description: St. George, Utah : Life Tumbled LLC, [2021] | Interest age level: 012-018. | Includes bibliographical references. | Summary: "Author Malissa Kelsch shares essential yet overlooked lessons she has picked up tumbling along life's many unexpected paths. Life Tumbled teaches Christian young women about: managing your money wisely; dating with an eternal perspective; achieving your potential through goal-setting; building your character to find joy within; developing your spiritual awareness to find peace; being industrious by gaining experience, competence, and skill; shaping ourselves after disappointment"--Provided by publisher.
    Identifiers: ISBN 9781737481706 (hardcover) | ISBN 9781737481713 (softcover) | ISBN 9781737481720 (ebook)
    Subjects: LCSH: Christian teenagers--Life skills guides--Juvenile literature. | Christian teenagers--Conduct of life--Juvenile literature. | Teenage girls--Religious life--Juvenile literature. | Teenage girls--Life skills guides--Juvenile literature. | Teenage girls--Conduct of life--Juvenile literature. | Christian life--Juvenile literature. | CYAC: Christian teenagers--Life skills guides. | Christian teenagers--Conduct of life. | Teenage girls--Religious life. | Teenage girls--Life skills guides. | Teenage girls--Conduct of life. | Christian life.
    Classification: LCC BV4551.3 .K45 2021 (print) | LCC BV4551.3 (ebook) | DDC 248.833--dc23

Special discounts for bulk sales are available.
Please contact malissa@lifetumbled.com.

For my dad, Roger William Osness Jr., because he taught me to face my fears and choose the grit that shaped my character. For my mother, Sally Ann, for always helping me see opportunities. For my husband, Keith, for sharing his love, persistence, and example. My kids, Kaden, Kyler, Makinzie, and Parker, who make life an adventure. My sister-in-law Kris Winkel for her matchmaking skills. Natalie, Ashley, Mike, Tami, Chelsea, Dorothy, and Melanie, who were my biggest cheerleaders for the book. Robin and Melissa for their special grit. My conglomerate of friends, family, and mentors who help smooth me out. Joshua, for the prepping and buffing of this book to shine.

Names have been changed to protect identities, and Emma is a combination of young women we have helped over the years. Maybe there is a part of you in Emma?

What if this is amazing?
What if this experience changes me for the better?
What if I grow?

—Mindy Gledhill

Be yourself; everyone else is taken.

—Oscar Wilde

Contents

What's Next? We Tumble Together!

www.LifeTumbled.com

Life is best lived with other people. Other people who believe as you believe. Other people who've been where you are. Other people who want the absolute best for you. If only you knew where to find them . . .

Well, you can! Head on over to my website where you'll find a newsletter, podcast, and community of other people to tumble along life's way with. We can't wait to meet you.

www.LifeTumbled.com

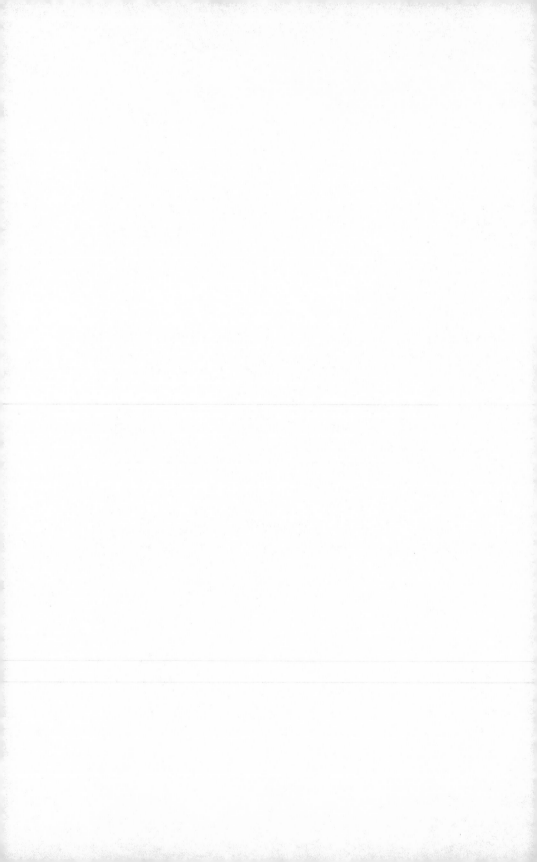

Tell Me What You Think

Let other readers know what you thought of *Life Tumbled*. Please write an honest review for this book on your favorite online bookshop.

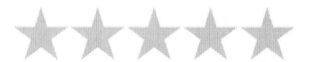

CHAPTER I

A Life Tumbled

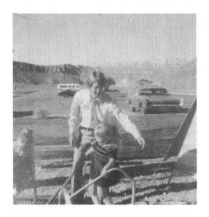

The man who moves a mountain begins by carrying away small stones.
—Confucius

On Sunday evening, August 12, 2001, my family was all together at my mom and dad's house for a birthday celebration for my sister-in-law. We always gathered on Sunday, but this time we were having dinner together too. Dad loved the kitchen and had prepared a signature dish—spaghetti with meat sauce—for the whole family that night. And he knew how to make food for a crowd with minimal messes. "Clean as you go," he always said.

There were eighteen of us at that time, with four of my siblings still living at home. My brothers would set up extra tables and chairs for all of us to be in the same room. We lined up the dishes at the lower counter for the kids to hang out and eat together. The food was set up on the island buffet style so everyone could go back for seconds. There were a few gifts for my sister-in-law on the table and a cake with not enough candles because after twenty-one, you never grow old.

After a full evening of laughing, visiting, and eating, it was time to go home. We always hug everyone goodbye when we leave the house. This time Keith, my husband, and I were distracted with our young children, ages six, five, and one, and didn't pause to give my dad a hug. I thought to myself, *I'll see him tomorrow and give him my hug then. No big deal.*

The very next day, my father was killed in an automobile accident on his way to work. A drunk driver hit him head-on on a quiet highway in another county. The driver had two passengers and two dogs. Everyone died; no one saw the accident. A big-rig truck driver came upon the accident and called it in. Through the transfer of information, the police officer who came to our family home got my dad's name wrong.

"You have the wrong house," my mother told the officer.

But when she called my dad's work, they said he had never showed. She called every fifteen minutes, hoping and praying. Still nothing. Around 6:00 p.m., the police returned to confirm what my mom already knew. Her sweetheart was gone.

Meanwhile, Keith and I were at home finishing up dinner and planning an activity as a family when the phone rang. My younger brother was calling to give me the news. I was speechless and had to ask him to repeat it three times. I could not believe it. I was in disbelief. I went numb. I got off the phone, and Keith and I loaded up the kids.

We rushed over to my mom's house to be there for support, not knowing what any of us were going to do. Friends and neighbors were already gathering, and as the word spread, they continued to pour into the home. I was in shock and still could not wrap my head around the situation. I tried to console my mom and tell her everything would be OK. We, your children, all seven of us, will help take care of you. My youngest brother was only twelve. I also have a special-needs sister who usually goes with Dad on work trips, but this time, she had stayed home.

We stayed up late. I remember calling all my dad's close friends and business partners to give them the news. Love poured in. My dad had touched so many lives, both within our family and in the community. At that time, he had been caring for his mother, who had lost Grandpa two years before to cancer. My dad visited every Monday to help pay her bills and drop off groceries. She loved visiting with her son. Now there would be yet another hole in her life.

My dad also took care of his sisters, nieces, nephews, and many friends and acquaintances. He had provided jobs to many over the years. He supported entrepreneurs just starting out and gave generously. He would stop at lemonade stands or stay up all night for fundraisers. He was loved by many.

At that time, my two boys and my daughter loved rockhounding. They would find rocks and bring them home. When we went on trips and local adventures, we would buy and gather rocks. We had quite a collection. A couple of months after my father's death, I bought an electric rock tumbler to polish the rocks. The instructions said to fill the barrel three-quarters full of stones, pour in the package of coarse grit provided, add water to just below the top of the stones, and then put on the lid. Run the tumbler for seven days, twenty-four hours a day, I read. After each seven-day period, clean out the barrel and repeat the process with a fine grit, prepolish, polish, and then a final detergent before the rocks would be finished. The instructions also said that the tumbler should be "burped" each day to relieve buildup of gas pressure.

I decided to set up and plug in our tumbler outside under the carport so we didn't have to hear it churn constantly. I began the process. After seven days of churning, I checked the rocks. The water, grit, and still-jagged rocks had formed a slurry mud together. I was surprised. The rocks were not ready for the next step. How long would this process take?

As I stood in my kitchen leaning over the barrel of rocks, I began to cry. I missed Dad. I still felt numb with him gone. He brought fun to this life. I took a deep breath to gather myself, and I felt my father's presence and heard his voice in my mind for the first time since his passing. His spirit told me this story.

Life on earth is like this rock tumbler. In our pre-earth life, our spirits have these beautiful colors. We come to earth and are born into a body of clay with our colorful personality and jagged edges to be shaped by experiences. Earth life tumbles us with all kinds of grit to wear down our sharp edges and shape our souls so our colors can shine. The other rocks help shape us too. When you bump up against another, it can help remove the jagged edges. You can choose people and experiences in your life to help shape you. Don't be afraid to learn and grow. Then my father's spirit whispered to me in a more courageous and adamant tone: *"If I knew what I know now, I would not be afraid. I would have done so much more. Do Good. Be not afraid. Go for it, Malissa!"* I felt at peace.

When a life is taken early (by early, I mean by our earthly standard), we feel great sadness. And we're reminded that none of us knows our day and time. The Lord has his own plan for us. It may not be what we wanted, but it is a *good* plan. As spirits, we are unable to be shaped into the beings Heavenly Father desires we become. Earthly life, these physical bodies, give us an incredible opportunity. We mustn't waste it. Unlike a video game, in which, when the avatar dies, it can regenerate, real life offers no do-overs. After death, we may want to try again. We may wish we could have done better, more, differently. But it's too late. And that is a regret I don't want to feel.

In nature, rocks are tumbled in streams, oceans, wind, and rain. I've written this book so you won't stay on the shoreline missing out on the opportunity to adventure as we tumble. No one can do it for you. You're giving this book a shot because in some ways (or many), it is for both of us. With the changing of time, becoming a self-sufficient adult can seem even more complicated. We are smack-dab in what feels like the slurry with our jagged edges. Still being churned with more to come.

I may not have all the answers, but I want to share with you my discoveries, the grit in my barrel that knocked off some of my jagged edges.

I've learned lessons around managing money wisely; dating with an eternal perspective; achieving my great potential through goal setting; building character to find joy within; developing spiritual awareness to find peace; and being industrious by gaining experience, competency, and skill. Being a mom now with three adult children, I want to pass these insights on to any daughter who needs them . . . even if you're not mine.

These foundational principles were pivotal discoveries in the process of being tumbled. If these answers are so important (they are), why did it take me so long to write this book? Well, we often take for granted our dreams, our bucket list ideas, because we know that one day will come when we have more time and energy. But something else always comes up, and we put off those dreams. One day, we'll get to them. But one day doesn't always come.

With this book, I'm giving my key moments that sent me tumbling so you can make the most of your one shot. You'll only be this age once. Everything you build now, you get to live off (or not) for the rest of your life. Decisions you make, skills you pick up, and wisdom you gather now determine your trajectory. It will be either a path of profound meaning or a path of confusion and disappointment.

I'm not promising a bed of roses, Prince Charming, or happily ever after. Sometimes, life teaches us through a barrel of rocks, grit, and water. These hard times shape and reveal the gem within the stone. There are many things to be afraid of in this world, but I do not want you to be afraid of the opportunities you see or may not see. The only thing to be afraid of is doing nothing. I hope you will see the possibilities and be excited about the opportunities you have.

This book is to remind us not to be afraid to gather people in our lives who encourage us, shape the jagged edges of our personalities, and wash our spirits with love to make us shine by saying, "*You got this!*" with the Lord cheering us on.

CHAPTER 2

Find Your Rocks: Growing Up Is Hard. Let's Make It an Adventure.

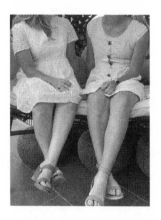

I am not afraid. I was born to do this.
—Joan of Arc

I'd like you to meet Emma. We live in the same neighborhood. She is every bit of eighteen years old. The first thing you'd notice is her curly, ripe, strawberry-red hair and her polka-dot glasses. You'd smile at Emma's pink cowgirl boots—and she'd smile back. Then she'd invite you to come along to whatever she's up to next. Expect a bubbly conversation. But not like the clear bubbles you blow off a wand. Those pop with the slightest breeze. Emma is resilient. Like bubble gum, you can chew for hours, but the fruity flavor never fades.

Emma knows what it's like to be blown and reblown like bubble gum. Pushed to the point at which she might pop. Over and over. Somehow, she keeps it together.

Emma's parents aren't church people. Emma wasn't either until school friends invited her to the church youth group in her neighborhood. It was either go or stay home and break up her divorcing parents' next bitter argument. She wanted some peace and quiet and figured church couldn't be any worse than home. So she went.

For the first time in her life, Emma found her own happy place. Somewhere she could let all that red hair down. Where people loved her for who she was. She was a new person in a Christian place, and if Christians are worth their salt, a new person is a treasure to welcome in and love. Emma attracted this new warmth. Her red hair alone was a hot commodity, something different to attract the very interested. She was luckily in a place she could learn the values her parents had failed to model.

Even though Emma's new church family accepted her, she felt like an outsider. She hadn't grown up learning the story of Lehi's family leaving Jerusalem, the reverence we show during sacrament, or a young woman's leadership potential within a church community. It turns out that the basic knowledge Emma lacked didn't matter as much as she thought it did. It all came together for her at General Conference.

One of the Elders was talking about his deceased wife, and he kept repeating, "Am I doing everything I can to hold her hand again?" She wrote down the phrase, thinking of her past boyfriend. However, after she wrote it down, she noticed she had written it as "Am I doing everything to hold His hand again?" She had capitalized the H in *his*. She automatically had a vividly clear image of Heavenly Father holding a little girl's hand. She knew she was that little girl. She didn't always know the right answer or do the right thing, but she did know that her life had a purpose. She was important to Him. The gospel of Jesus Christ taught her that she had a purpose, and that knowledge is helping her soul find peace, joy, and the essence of her potential. All our potential.

Emma had finally caught a glimpse of what meaningful relationships could be like. She had found a group of people she could go to who had answers to life's most important questions and wanted her own family to experience it as well. Of course, she did! She felt like what she had found could repair her parents' relationship, bring the family together, and make life enjoyable. If only she could bring them toward these truths.

As she looked back, however, she realized it was the perfect circumstance for her. Families in her ward (community church members) had all but adopted Emma as their own daughter, their own sister, giving her in many ways what she needed but didn't get from home. She witnessed many people serving each other and finding joy in that loving service. Her Young Women leaders welcomed her by immediately including her in an event they were putting together that showcased each girl and their individual talents. They worked with Emma to find out more about her, what she dreamed of becoming, and what brought her joy. These were questions no one had ever asked her before. They discovered she loved horses and art. One of the leaders let her borrow a beautiful dress and jewelry for the special evening. She felt like a beautiful daughter loved for her unique talents and abilities. In class at church, she learned about the industriousness of service and how it brings joy to engage in good causes. She deepened her understanding of love and eternal perspective. Besides learning the purpose of life, she learned many of life's hacks dealing with others. She began to understand how her family dealt with contention and how it was possible to handle disagreements or hurt in a different manner with love.

When Emma first entered the Young Women's program for our church, she wanted her family to join her church too. That didn't happen. In fact, her home life got worse after she started going to church. Her parents' strife became too much to handle. She was glad to have a place of refuge, but she needed out of her unsafe situation.

In the middle of her senior year, Emma moved out to live with a family she met at church—us! Yes, young Emma became our new roommate. This provided a gradual transition into the real world. She had a safety net, which felt even safer when her mom passed away from aggressive cancer, and her father turned to alcohol as a way to deal with loss.

Even before moving out and losing her mom, Emma had felt lost and was searching for answers. She didn't know how to "adult," but she wanted to. (Think the big things in life, like how to find a genuine, caring, loyal husband and grow together as teammates and be friends.) She wanted to learn all the simple things like cooking pancakes, scrambling eggs, and preparing boxed lunches to go.

We took Emma on a road trip once. We packed healthy snacks of carrots, celery, granola bars, grapes, crackers, and cheese. She had never thought of packing her own food because her parents always bought fast food or grabbed something at the gas station. They never planned what to eat—they never planned anything.

A lot of young women are like Emma. Maybe your mom and dad raised you well, but they had a limited view of the world, and you want to understand how other people have been raised. You have realized that your parents may not know everything. Maybe you've promised yourself you will *not* turn out like your mother. Perhaps you have not had a mother to rely on to ask questions or receive guidance from. Perhaps, like Emma, your mom failed to lead by example or is no longer in the picture.

In many ways, you see yourself in Emma. I see parts of my story in hers too. When I graduated from high school, my family moved away from me to another state. I had to grow up really fast. I moved in with my best friend, Kerri, and her family and started college. A few months into school, Kerri got engaged, and I needed to move out. I was scared and didn't know what I was going to do. My parents could not sell their house, so we came up with a plan for me to move in and take over paying the mortgage. I had to put the utilities in my name, get a washer and dryer, and find roommates to help pay the mortgage. I was eighteen and felt really alone trying to handle all this adulting. I had to become an independent woman. This was my first big transition into adulthood—I was stepping into a new barrel to be tumbled with the grit of real life. Stepping out on my own was shaping me into a person who could survive—and thrive. I didn't know it then, but I would find out that life was going to smooth me over and bring out my shine.

CHAPTER 3

Jump in the Barrel: How to Set and Achieve Any Goal

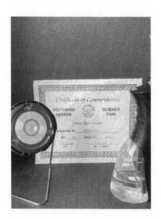

The secret of getting ahead is getting started.
—Mark Twain

It was the first day of school. I could smell the new jeans and sharpened pencils. The excitement of having a new backpack. The large stack of books for class. Both still felt light.

The high school halls were all outdoors and encircled an atrium. There were a few loud, goofy students, but for the most part, everyone was trying not to look lost as they found their classes.

I was on my way to third period. Science. It was always the hardest class. How would I pass? Would I need a tutor? Would I sit by smart people who could help me? What if I failed? My 3.75 GPA would drop significantly. Then how would I get college scholarships?

I walked into class and saw my science teacher for the first time. Mr. Smith. A tall, slender man with a slight pot belly. His white button-down shirt was tucked into black polyester pants. His black hair was combed in front with a slight dishevel in the back.

He welcomed everyone to class in a soft-spoken voice. He let us choose which cold stainless-steel table we wanted to sit at. "Four to a table, please," he mumbled. I sat in the second row in the back, away from the door. A few stoners and band students sat near me. We were slightly more than acquaintances; we took physics class together.

Mr. Smith handed out our syllabi and went over the rules, supplies needed, and class outline. He told us about the science fair that would be held in the spring. He announced that all who wanted to participate would get extra credit.

"Whoever wins first place at the school science fair and first place at regionals will get an automatic A in the class for the year," Mr. Smith added.

That's it! I thought. *I will win the science fair to get my A.*

I would need help. There, at the start of class, I began devising my plan. A family friend came to mind. Dennis, a college student, liked science. I figured I could ask him for help.

That very weekend, I ran over to Dennis's house and asked if he would help me with my science project.

"Be glad to," Dennis said.

Yes!

For weeks, Dennis and I brainstormed ideas. By October, we'd narrowed it down to a project that would prove the equation of gravity. Supplies for the demonstration were readily available, and we had a variety of ways we could do it and look pretty cool.

To prove gravity, we used a garden hose first, to watch the water flow out and fall to the ground. Then I went to a waterpik water flosser since it's smaller and can squirt water out in a tight space. My dad had helped me build a fully enclosed six-by-four-by-three-foot wooden box, which we painted black. We cut a slit in the front so an observer could peek inside the box and watch the experiment take place. To help with the visual, I tacked string to make a grid on the inside back wall and added a strobe light to capture the water droplets in motion as they fell. We graphed the path of the water and put the numbers in the equation to prove gravity.

That A is mine, I thought.

By the science fair in February, I was more than ready. I showed up at 8:00 a.m. on the dot in a dress that looked professional. I was excused from classes to demonstrate my project and let the judges ask questions. When the first judge stopped at my booth, I explained my project. He bent over to look through the slit, and I started the strobe light and the waterpik. I hadn't noticed that the waterpik was turned slightly toward the front—a result of transporting my exhibit, I guess—and it shot water right into the judge's eyes. I was mortified, but the judge just laughed. By noon, all the judging was complete. I figured my worst fear would come true. I did all this work, I had one shot, and my grade currently hovered right above a D because I was not a good test taker.

I was a nervous wreck for the rest of the day. The school winners would be announced at 9:00 a.m. Science class was at 10:00 a.m. When the loudspeaker crackled, I stopped breathing. First came earth science. Then chemistry. Then my category, physics. I didn't make it to third place. Or second. I thought my heart would stop.

"And in first place, Malissa Osness."

What? I did it? I won?

I immediately returned to life.

That A was all but mine! If my school's judges loved my project, surely the regional judges would too.

I jumped up and down and could hardly concentrate the entire hour before science. I bounced into class to the applause and cheers of my classmates. Then Mr. Smith joined us, announced the top three again for physics, and congratulated me. Now I just had to win the regional science fair.

On a sunny day in March, I was excused to participate. I showed up dressed for success. But when I brought in my giant black box, I got looks. Some curious. Others dismissive. I, too, had my doubts. This was going to be tough. There were really smart people there. The sort of people who get As the normal way. At least I didn't squirt anyone in the eye. I learned that lesson the first time.

At the end of the long day, we listened for the results. Third place, then second were announced back to back.

"Placing first in physics, Malissa Osness!"

The official might as well have said, "With an A in physics, Malissa Osness!" Because that's what I heard. By then, my grade in the class had dropped to a D—failure—but first place wiped my slate clean.

Back in class the next day, Mr. Smith congratulated me.

"But I can't just give you an A, Malissa," he then said. "I can't fix all your other work."

"What?" I screeched.

My classmates gasped.

"But you promised!" someone shouted.

"Yeah, how is that fair?" said another.

"The school district really wouldn't approve this." Mr. Smith shrugged. "I just assumed that a student with a passing grade already would win."

"But you didn't say that," I said.

The class backed me up. Uproars continued.

"All right, all right!" Mr. Smith waved us quiet. "Fine, Malissa can have her A. Can we please just get back to class? We've got a lot of material to cover today."

You've never seen someone smirk so big.

I got my A.

I was happy.

This is the point of my story: every goal has many paths to success. Many times we think there is only one way to get things done, but often, life's toughest challenges bring with them several opportunities to overcome them as long as you know how to look for them. Just because something is laid out to be achieved in one way doesn't mean that's the only way to accomplish it. In fact, as you creatively reconsider what you think is possible, you may realize that by accomplishing one goal, you can accomplish many goals.

One Goal to Achieve Them All

In 2003, the tables had turned. Now I was the teacher. At the time, I was a working mother who counseled underprivileged high schoolers. It was my job to help these kids find their own path to success in a world that hadn't handed them many clear opportunities.

One day, a student came to my office to go over options for merit scholarships. He mentioned that he had finished the Saint George Marathon that past year. Wow. I was impressed. He was not in the best shape, nor was I back then. I imagined marathon runners as tall and lean; this boy was short and pudgy. Yet he had completed the marathon with such a good time, he received a medal. This got me thinking.

If he can do it, I can too. And I will.

As soon as the student left my office, I googled "How do you run a marathon?" because I didn't have the first clue. Apparently, before you complete a marathon, you have to train. That seemed obvious enough. Does that mean running every day? Hiking on the weekend? Walking a lot? Doing some stretches in the morning? Internet searches answered these and other questions, but the problem was that there were too many strategies. What was the right path for me as a beginner? So I took my study offline—that night, I reached out to a friend I recalled running every morning before work.

"I run five miles a day," she told me over the phone.

"That sounds like a lot," I said.

"It takes me an hour, yeah."

"An *hour*? You run for a whole *hour*? How can you run for an hour? Don't you get tired? And bored?"

"No, it's stress relieving, actually. It's my time out in nature. When I start, it's dark outside, and by the time I'm done, the sun is rising. It makes me feel really good."

I'd heard of the runner's high. This must be what she was describing.

I couldn't commit to go the whole five miles, but because I'd already told myself I would run that marathon, I had to do *something*. I had found a beginner's guide to running a marathon, which recommended starting with one mile.

So that's what I did. On my first day of training, I got up at 4:30 a.m., met my friend at the curb, walked up a steep hill, and ran to the stop sign and back. A couple of hundred yards round trip. Just the warm-up walking up the hill was enough for me.

The next week, I continued to run with my friend. Every morning, we warmed up by walking up the hill, then we started our run down the street past the stop sign, around the neighborhood, and back. The week after, even farther. I kept going until I could run a full mile without stopping. Several months later, I could join my friend for three of her five miles. She would run ahead to get her five miles in and catch up with me on her way back so we ended together. During one run, I talked her into joining me for the marathon. She was so much faster; I thought she could definitely complete the marathon.

Spring came, and it was time to register. Now the real fun began. A 26.2-mile marathon would not train itself. We had to take baby steps. We had our running schedule, and we were as consistent as two moms with jobs could be. We ran at five o'clock every morning and, on Saturdays, took a long run around town. It wasn't easy. We had to take running routes that had bathrooms along the way. For some reason, my body was running on the inside too. We had to learn to run in the dark and not get hit by cars. After our long runs on Saturday, we would be sore for days, making it difficult to walk or go up stairs.

The first Saturday in October came—race day. We had to be on the bus at 5:00 a.m. to travel to the start line. We arrived with multiple layers of clothing, MP3 players, and fanny packs stuffed with energy snacks and aspirin.

At the start line, it was bitterly cold. Race volunteers gave us paper-thin blankets that looked like tin foil to help us retain body heat. We waited by a warm bonfire and listened to music on loudspeakers. The race would start promptly at 7:00 a.m., right at sunrise.

Every three miles, they told us, there would be a rest station with water, Gatorade, menthol cream for sore muscles, and a port-a-potty.

I started near the back of the pack. I didn't want to feel the pressure to run fast. I just wanted to finish; I didn't want to face the embarrassment of being picked up by the bus. That was the last hope of everyone who didn't train and thought they didn't have to or got injured. That would *not* be me. As long as I followed a four-hour pace, I'd make it with plenty of time to spare.

The race was hard and beautiful. Volunteers offered relief and encouragement. By mile eighteen, I asked myself, *Why am I doing this?* I had to stop at every rest station. My friend had probably finished before I reached halfway. I couldn't even keep up with the four-hour pace. But I kept going.

The last mile was the hardest. I could see the finish line, but I was so tired. All I could do was put one foot in front of the other. It probably would have been faster to walk than trying to run.

Crossing the finish line was a relief. It was *over*. Other runners cheered. A volunteer put a medal around my neck and guided me to an area with food and first aid. I lay on the grass and took in deep breaths. *I did it! Wow! I really did it!*

What's the point of this marathon story? That marathons are really hard? Yes, that's one point. In goal setting, if you choose one big goal that by achieving it you achieve several other important goals, go for it. I had wanted to get back into shape. So I picked the one goal—training for a marathon—that would result in me eating healthy, getting active, feeling more energized, having more strength, and making new friends.

Setting the marathon goal was superior to counting calories at mealtime or joining a gym and being bored out of my mind on the treadmill. Marathon training gave me a goal, a deadline, and an accountability partner.

Two years passed between my initial desire to get fit and the marathon training. Other goals have taken me longer. They may for you too. And that's OK. What matters is getting all the right elements in place so you have a system to achieve your goal.

For nineteen years, I've wanted to write a book. It wasn't until I was in a car accident that I realized what I would regret not sharing if I died. This book would be my biggest regret if I left it unwritten. So how was I to achieve this goal of writing a book? I look at myself as an artist more than a writer. Over the years, I have had people say they would help me, but everyone was so nice or ended up being too busy. The question I asked myself was what I needed to do to accomplish this goal. I needed help. Just like with the science project, I needed someone who had gone before to guide me and hold me accountable. So I hired an editor and accountability partner, and I paid him! Nothing hurts more than losing money and, for me, not following through on a promise. And the fact that you're reading this book now proves it worked.

Whenever I first consider any goal, I write it at the top of a page in a notebook. If it is a big goal, I rip out the page and tape it to the wall so I can see it straight on. Once it's up there, I get sticky notes, write down every thought that comes to my mind about how to reach that goal, and stick them to the wall. As soon as I start to see similar tasks, I group those thoughts together. Then I organize them in order. I ask myself which ones are doable and which ones I need to find someone to help me with. At times, I think I can do it all, but often, when time and money will allow, it's better to have a professional help me out. If during the brainstorming process I get stuck, I put myself in a different environment to open up my creative process. I take a break and go for a walk, hike, or workout. When I come back to the challenge, I have fresh eyes. Most of the time, I find books or listen to podcasts. I stir up conversations in person or on social media for insight.

Once all the ideas are out, I set my plan of action. When is the best time to work on it? That's a good question—when should you work on *your* goal? If you are a morning person, set aside time to work on it before the distractions of the day push their way through. If you have to wake up an hour earlier to achieve your goal . . . do it. It will be worth it. When I was a teenager, my sister would get up at 5:00 a.m. to practice her violin. I could not figure out how she could do that. I loved my sleep. Now I get up at 5:00 a.m. myself because I feel motivated to achieve my goals. My husband is a night person, so that's when he works on his projects. I'll drag myself to bed, and he keeps on working.

Morning or night, set time aside to work on your goal consistently: daily, weekly, or monthly. Consistency prevents distraction. I have found progressing toward my goal at my own pace, as long as I keep it in focus, will get me where I want to be even if I am going it alone and have no externally imposed deadline. I always keep the meta goal in mind—the one big goal that, when achieved, results in many other successes. And you can too. Even if you don't have an accountability partner or external deadline, you'll be able to stay focused and consistent. If you have a goal with a deadline, you are more likely to accomplish it. So work toward your goal at the same time for the same amount of time until it's done. And it will be. Sooner than you think.

See? Goals aren't that hard after all. Just put one foot in front of the other.

CHAPTER 4

Bring On the Grit: How to Face the Real World

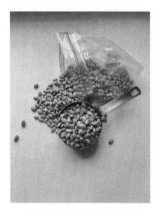

Expectation is the root of all heartache.
—William Shakespeare

When my two sons were small and I was pregnant with my daughter, we lived in northern Utah. I would commute an hour every day to the University of Utah and an hour home. I was gone for eleven to twelve hours each weekday. I was also the primary president at this time. My husband was teaching at the local high school. Being educators, we both had to work to make ends meet. My husband fell ill during this time. He was passing out several times a week. One night, he passed out in the bathroom against the door, and I could not get in to help him. I sat on the floor crying and praying he would be OK, that he would wake up from his fall and not be injured. We went to doctor after doctor and many specialists. No one could figure out what to do. With the medical bills rising and us missing work, our income was lower than our bills. We were having a really hard time financially. We never went out to eat or spent money frivolously. I would cook from scratch to make the budget go further.

Growing up in a church, I was told if I did everything right, including what was asked of me, we would be taken care of, so I happily paid my tithe. I always agreed to every calling, big or small. We gave of our time, talents, and whatever means we could to follow the gospel principles and the leaders.

During this hard time, my husband approached the bishop to ask for help because both our extended families were in dire straits themselves. My dad was out of work, and my husband's father barely had enough to keep his business afloat. We did what we had been taught to do when growing up: asked the church for help. We have a hard time asking for help. It's not in our nature when we feel we are smart and capable, but we had no food at this time. I recall a little flour, sugar, spices, tortillas in the fridge, and a bag of beans. I would soak the beans and make chili or refried beans for burritos to last for that evening and the next night's dinner.

When my husband asked the bishop for assistance, the bishop asked if we were full tithe payers. My husband replied yes. The bishop told my husband that was unusual. People who paid their tithing didn't have problems like this. We received no food assistance. At the same time, while I was at home, the Relief Society president called me to see if I could take a meal to a sick lady in the ward. I told her I had no food. I only had a bag of beans to feed my family. She said, "OK, we will get you next time" and hung up.

I felt despair. *How are we going to get through this?*

Let me make a point that if this had not happened to me personally, I would not have believed it. The church we belong to is very generous. I don't think these individuals really understood what we were asking for. This was a strong lesson that bad things happened to good people.

The next day, we heard a knock on the door and opened up to our neighbors, who did not practice our faith. They said hello, and I saw their car backed up in our driveway. They turned and started unloading food from the trunk of their car. I was amazed and asked, "How did you know we needed food?"

She said she had a feeling, and they were happy to do something for us.

As days passed, I began to get angry at the people in our church family. We go to church faithfully and pay tithes. We got married in the temple. We always had callings. I had served in the youth organization and then the children's program in the church. I had followed all the rules, and then the church was not there for us. A few more months passed, and I asked to be released from serving in the children's organization. The anger grew. I was thinking about leaving the church. All my life, I had been a devout member because I wanted to believe that the church was perfect, and if I just followed all the checklists, my life would be good.

One day at work, I told my story to a friend, a fellow member. She could tell I was angry. I told her I didn't care if I ever went back to church. I was done. She gave me great insight into the fact that even though the people at church were not there for me, the Lord was. The Lord knew what my family needed and had whispered our needs to my neighbor, who was listening. The Lord loves you. Find ways to see Him in your life. Find what the gospel of Jesus Christ really means to you. The culture of churches is laced with humans who are imperfect. I learned that people in the church will disappoint us, but the gospel truths remain true.

This is when I began searching fervently to understand what the gospel of Jesus Christ really means, not what I'm marking off the checklist in order to get to heaven. The Lord needed to grind my jagged edges of tradition away to be able to shape me with gospel truths. I also learned how to forgive and communicate more clearly.

I thought the culture of my church was the gospel. I had expectations and felt entitled. I discovered that my expectations were not truth centered, and I had created a fairy-tale type of life in my mind that certainly disappointed me. I'm sharing all this with you to help you guard your heart from disappointment and give you the courage to be strong in truth. I hope you will be conscious of your actions and not just follow blindly. It's OK to ask questions, knowing that Christ is the center. You need that connection. I have found there is no reason to be a skeptic or antagonistic. It's about my relationship with Christ and what is true. If you and others in the group are looking out for each other, and you're in it together, you'll blossom in a way you won't if you're in a bad environment. In order to love your neighbor as yourself, you need neighbors. And to love yourself if the neighbors don't, set realistic expectations of them and everyone else in your life.

At a certain age, every young woman asks herself, *Is reality ever going to live up to happily ever after?* Nowadays, women watch HGTV and expect their future husbands to renovate the bathroom on a weekend for $500! What kind of expectations and treatment of a relationship can this lead to? I think the reason the movie *Shrek* is so well loved is that it shows us that real life is not always a fairy tale.

My expectations of my future husband changed after I met Keith, and we married. Before that relationship, I had three non-negotiables about married life:

1. I will *not* live in Utah.
2. I will *not* work for family.
3. I will *never* live in a small town.

When I got married, I was going to UNLV, and Keith was graduating with his master's degree, so we got an apartment in Las Vegas. I had a good job and scholarships that would pay for my academics.

It was hot and horrible for Keith that summer, working outdoors in Las Vegas while trying to find work with his degree, so he started looking in other states, and Utah was on the list. His parents lived in Sterling and ran the oldest bed-and-breakfast in the state. There was a small junior college two towns away, and he applied for a teaching position there. He got the job, so we moved to Sterling, Utah, a town of two hundred, and we helped out at the family bed-and-breakfast. I learned real quick never to say never on variables that were not core values.

When we moved to Sterling, I gave up my scholarships to UNLV and wondered how I would finish my education. Blessed by the Lord, I got to be in the first group of students when Utah State University started trying out distance learning. They happened to have a small scholarship to help pay for a portion of my tuition each year. Two years later, I graduated with my degree in education. It was weird at the time never to set foot on campus until it was time to graduate.

We all fall or get knocked off the "how it's supposed to be" trajectory at some point in our lives. Even those who appear to have it all, those who "did everything right," will experience hardship. In my denomination, doing everything right means going to church, following the word of wisdom, and marrying a returning missionary in the temple.

If you don't follow the plan, are you still a good person? Yes! There are good people all around. Find the true motive of a person's heart, and you will see who they really are. Life is going to take us on our own path. Yes, those guidelines are a good measure, but the motive is the better measure. What is in your heart?

Even if the good things you expect to happen to you don't, all isn't lost. You always have the power within to change your circumstances. And you have the choice to exercise that power, evaluate what's really important to you, and build a beautiful life no matter what.

Will you?

CHAPTER 5

Change the Grit: How to Be a Good Kid When You're Not a Child Anymore

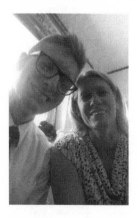

To be good, and do good, is the whole duty of man comprised in a few words.
—Abigail Adams

My oldest son and first to leave home went on his mission when he was nineteen. He was called for twenty-four months to the Melbourne, Australia, mission. He had the pleasure of serving with two mission presidents, and I had the joy of watching him grow. At the time, missionaries were permitted to call home twice a year, on Mother's Day and at Christmas. Throughout those other long months, Kaden kept in contact with us through once-a-week emails and the occasional letter. He endured experiences I could not have imagined going through myself, and worse, he was going through them without any support from his parents. For example, he lived in the roughest area of a town out in the bush. He had personal belongings stolen repeatedly. Others out in the mission field sabotaged his efforts, knowingly or absentmindedly. All things considered, my son left as a teenage boy and was about to return as a young man.

I was so excited for him to come home in June at the conclusion of his two years of service. I made all the necessary arrangements—getting his room ready, letting family know when to come visit, setting up school and job opportunities, all the logistical readjustments.

When I didn't get word on when Kaden's flight home would touch down, I called the mission home in Melbourne.

"Didn't he tell you?" the mission president's assistant asked me.

"Tell me? Tell me what?" I panicked.

"Because there's a new incoming mission president, Kaden has the option to stay on for one more transfer. He accepted."

"One more transfer?"

"Yes, for six weeks."

I was shocked. And mad. Kaden hadn't asked his own mother if he could stay out longer on his mission. Then I realized . . . he didn't have to. He didn't have to tell me. Kaden was an adult. He could make that decision for himself.

What a feeling to be a mother for twenty-one years and finally step back to let my child fly. Don't take me for one of those really controlling mothers. I've raised my kids to know the truth and given them opportunities to exercise their free agency. But that moment woke me up to the fact that my oldest, just like me, was an adult.

It's a strange season for both sides when the child becomes an adult. All these years of helping and guiding, and now we're on the sidelines of their lives to be there if or when we are needed.

Using the "life tumbled" analogy, it's like being in the first tumbling process with the large grit to shape us. We grind for years, maybe eighteen, maybe twenty-one. Our parents bump us and shape us. Then one day, we look in the tumbler and realize it's time to be put in with a different grit, finer, to really shape us. It's tricky to know when that is. Most of the time, it's the transition of moving out of our parents' home. Some of us may be afraid that we won't be able to make it on our own and will have to come back to our parents'. Others are ready for the adventure. I felt both.

When I was fourteen years old, I struggled with my mother. I was sensitive. I felt criticized and unappreciated for the things I did around the house. I had five younger siblings, and there was a lot to do, tend, and clean. One day, I'd had enough. I ran away. I felt I was smart enough to get along on my own. So I packed a bag and took off. I knew my parents would look for me at my best friend's home, so I bounced around for a few hours. I hung out with a friend from the bus stop because my parents wouldn't know to call there.

Finally, when it got dark, I went to my best friend's house. That was probably the only place I could have spent the night. She let me stay, and my dad found me by phone. I was willing to speak with him, but not Mom.

"You need to come home."

"I'm not living with Mom!"

"Your mother loves you. She cares about you," Dad said.

"I know, but I just don't want to be doing any more work. I'm ready to go out on my own."

"Let's give it one more try. Stay the night there with your friend, and we'll be ready for you to come home in the morning. We love you, and we need you in this family."

I knew he was right. My family needed me. My younger siblings needed me. My mom needed me. That night as I drifted off to sleep at my best friend's, I thought about how hard she had it. A stay-at-home mom responsible for seven children. Her oldest was busy with work, school, and dating, and that left only her and me to take care of five children, three of whom were needy toddlers. Dad and Mom were my biggest cheerleaders. And I realized my mom needed some cheering herself. My youngest siblings would soon be all grown up like my older sister. Being Mom's assistant wouldn't last forever, or even much longer. Soon I'd be off living my own life, and she would be alone at home with five children.

Mom needed me.

I had to get home.

I got up at dawn, ran home, snuck in through the back door, cleaned the bathroom, and diapered the baby.

I now realize I needed my parents just as much as they needed their little rebellious fourteen-year-old. I felt strong, like I could venture out on my own. But I, too, needed a safety net. Roaming around the neighborhood for those few hours before talking to my dad, I had no clue what to do with myself. How in the world could I have figured out where to live, how to get a job, and what to cook for myself, all while trying to salvage relationships I'd ruined with heartbroken parents and siblings who missed me?

If it's time to move out for your own personal safety, then by all means, go. At least look before you leap. Plan better than I did. Surround yourself with wise counsel from adults you respect and trust. If you don't have to leave home immediately but you know it's in your near future, use this time to explore and build more strength with opportunities in work. Work is a way to get out of the house and learn to be an adult.

That's what I did. I got a part-time job a few weeks after ending my runaway journey early. The job gave me an opportunity to make my own money, survive on my own when it was time to move out at age eighteen, and earn more respect from my mother. *Wow, my daughter is growing up and taking on more responsibility.* This also relieved her of the pressure of providing for some of my needs. It built my confidence because I could pick out the clothes I wanted, even if they cost more than the family budget would have allowed. Looking good helped me feel better about myself.

While I was out of the house working, my mother was figuring out how to make it through the day with five kids and one fewer pair of hands to help. There is a family shift that occurs when someone leaves the house to work or get married. I had to have as much empathy for my mother as I expected her to have for me. She had it harder than I had been willing to admit to myself. That's why I stayed. And why I did my chores. Because my mom was human too.

I remember the day my son realized that his parents were not perfect. He said that growing up, we were his heroes. We were having a conversation at home, and Keith stated a fact. Later, Kaden realized that there was another perspective, and in his eyes, his dad was not correct this time. It crushed him to know his dad was not perfect, but it gave him the first step to start to think on his own and ask more questions. Now when he wonders about something, he studies and searches for answers. He asks for advice, but in the end, he has to make the decision. This is a transition that has to happen to all of us. We all need to study and discover answers on our own.

Everyone is doing the best they can with the knowledge and experience they have at that moment. A word of warning: you have your free agency. Use it wisely. Choose good, honorable people to tumble with now that you're out of your parents' barrel and on your own. Build valuable relationships with people who do good in the world, who respect you, and who clearly want the best for you. These can be friends, mentors, colleagues, roommates, or fellow believers. In short, make friends with people who will help and inspire you. That also means avoiding people whose lives you don't want yours to resemble—people whose choices result in addiction, substance abuse, financial ruin, dysfunctional relationships, and even crime.

Friends will help shape your perspective and attitude. After all, you are the sum of the five people you associate with most closely. Who is influencing you? Do you have mentors who will lift you? We women need each other. We need conversation. We need to bounce ideas and express ourselves. It relieves stress. I have found it of great importance since I got married to have a good group of friends who will uplift, inspire, and encourage me with my dreams. Having the right friends to help you grow in truth will keep you on the bright side of life. If you hang out with people who think the world is out to get them, their unhelpful belief can hold *you* back. When you get married, you will still need friends because our nature is to give, and we need an outlet to remember who we are as individuals. Friends who help you grow are as essential to your health as vitamins.

The best way to honor your parents now that you're your own person is by being an independent adult who doesn't need Dad and Mom to make good decisions for you—because you can do that yourself.

CHAPTER 6

Tumble Along: How to Save Money, Move Out, and Live Like an Adult

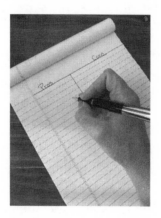

The price of greatness is responsibility.
—Winston Churchill

When I graduated high school at eighteen and started my first year of college, my family had an opportunity to move back to Utah. In my mind, I had always expected to move away from my family. I thought I would be the adventurous one and leave home on my own terms. Here I was, now faced with the reality of being left on my own to grow up. *Wow. How am I going to do this? I have school and work. Where will I live?* The thought of paying rent was an eye-opener.

Luckily, my mom had taught me how to save money, so I had a little nest egg to survive for a couple of months. Also, like Emma, I had a friend whose family let me live with them for a few months. As time passed, my parents could not sell their home, which put them in a stressful situation. They could not afford to keep paying two mortgages, so we came up with a plan. I would live in the house, get roommates, and pay the mortgage. I quickly went to work to make this plan happen. I put an advertisement up at the Institute of Religion for roommates, and word began to spread. It wasn't long before the shared rooms filled up, which left one private room available. It was more expensive, and I needed it filled. I did feel some relief that most of the mortgage and utilities would be paid. I could work extra hours to make up the difference, but I really needed to fill the last room, and by miracles, that person would change the rest of my life.

I was adulting. The grit of life was quickly shaping me in this area. It took great courage on all our parts. The thought of my parents turning over a house, one of the biggest investments of their lives, to a fresh adult who knew pretty much nothing about living on her own, paying bills, or maintaining a house. I still felt like a kid who wanted to be an adult but just got thrown into the real world.

I was blessed to have parents who believed in me and felt more confidence in my abilities than I had myself. They had plenty on their mind with the move and five children still at home. They definitely didn't have time to micromanage me. They did, however, have the faith to let me work out most of the details on my own. I put the utilities in my name, found a used washer and dryer that were within my budget, and was able to pay the mortgage. My parents have seen me take on hard things and trusted I could figure it out. And I did.

These transitions into adulthood can be awkward and really hard. I have seen many different situations of people moving out and being independent. Be patient and honorable with yourself and your parents. There will be many discoveries throughout this process. And some may not go the way you expected. Seek authentic ways to build genuine relationships. Some parents micromanage or helicopter their children. Just respectfully reconfirm to them how great they did in raising you. They want you to succeed, but it may be unfamiliar territory for them too.

We have had many people live with us over the years during their transitioning into an independent adult. The boys from Colorado City who lost their family, home, culture, religion, and town. Many students, family, and even homeless couples lived with us for a short time. There are all kinds of stories and transitions. One young lady who lived with us had her mom come and help her move in. She got settled in, and the mother stayed for a week. The young lady had just graduated college and gotten a job in our town. Her parents were glad for her to have a new environment to help her grow. Like some parents, though, they had a hard time recognizing her strength and championing her independence.

It's tough as a parent to see your child fall. Inadvertently, we create safety nets, just in case the child stumbles. This young lady started off well and was excited about her independence. We watched her bounce back and forth with her confidence about being able to make it on her own. She would have good days and bad days. One day she confided in me that her mom had done a lot for her, and she hadn't taken the opportunity to work beside her mom on many daily chores because her mom could do them so quickly and make things look so good. She didn't want to mess up and was afraid of doing the little things wrong. She wanted to be like her mom and other women she knew and felt were accomplished. I had her take a deep breath and realize they had once been in her shoes too. I told her to enjoy this moment where she was and take one thing at a time. "You will get there. You will learn through experience and by trying over and over again. Enjoy each moment as you tumble along."

Another choice she had to make while she was with us was whether or not to change jobs. She was very loyal and committed to her first job. A friend had gotten her an opportunity for a higher paying job, but it was part commission. Her friend was doing well at the job, but she was afraid she was not as outgoing. She didn't realize her sweet disposition and great listening skills would have helped her do well. She didn't take the job because of her fear of failing.

The first thing I always tell people that have choices to make is to create a pros-and-cons list. Write it out so you can see it on paper outside your head. For some reason, the mind will hold on to the emotional part and make something bigger than it needs to be when it is not written down. Currently, I have a client who is afraid to move. Her husband has a job out of state and has to commute for ten hours every weekend to come home. He wants her to sell the house, but she is afraid of being homeless because homes are so expensive, even though she does not need a big house anymore. She could get a newer, smaller house with less upkeep and be near her grandkids. Her fear is holding her back. I don't know all the details, but I have asked her to make a list and write out the pros and cons so her emotions can shift if they need to. Instead of focusing on fear of what she is giving up, she can see in writing what she is getting and get excited instead of afraid. Satan wants us to be afraid. He does not want us to grow and progress.

Responsibility helps you grow up fast. As soon as you take on responsibility, that's when you gain competency, wisdom, and experience. How much responsibility do you want to take on? Remember, once you take it on, there's no off-loading it. Your eyes have been opened. Sometimes you want to run backward, but in the long run, it's always better to adopt responsibility than dismiss it.

The biggest concerns most people have when they become adults is where they're going to live. Should they move out now? What are their options?

Renting an apartment can be beneficial when you are just starting out and don't know your true direction. It gives you the opportunity to look in other areas for employment if the job you have does not work out. We bought a home in Tooele when we probably should have rented. Keith got a job teaching at the local high school, and he did not like it. He was used to college- and university-level teaching, and the job actually made him sick. He ended up quitting and going back to Snow College, and we had to figure out how to sell or rent the home. We decided to rent and had great renters at first, but the second family destroyed the home. We ended up having to put more money into it to sell it, and the rent we received over the years didn't even cover the mortgage, so we were going in the hole keeping the home. If we had just rented and tried out the job and the area, we could have left without all the stress and struggle. We'd bought the house because we thought we were behind in life. At our age, we should have a home. That's the American dream. Sometimes it's OK to wait and just rent.

Let's talk about the other options for moving out. It all depends on how responsible you want to be. Responsibility is a choice. If you only plan on staying in the town you're living in for a short time, then the options can include renting a room or a studio apartment. If you are going to school, do you want to live on campus and have the college life or off campus, which may allow you to save money by cooking your own food. What kind of experience do you want to have, and what is your budget? Just starting out, I would suggest you live as cheaply as possible to save your money and invest in yourself for school or long-term goals like buying a car, buying a house, or starting a business. Word of warning: don't spend a large sum for a car. It will be a waste of money. Cars are an expenditure, not an asset. Be conservative so you can save.

My observation has been that the more you live alone, the more you get stuck in your own ways. We were meant to bump up against each other in life. I encourage you to find a roommate or two—or more. When you live with others, you not only save money; you also have fun, learn how to get along, and pick up unexpected skills. With five roommates, I quickly learned how to ask for what I needed or wanted, how to pay bills, and how to honor people's privacy. I learned to be patient and work around schedules, especially with laundry and bath-room time. I also discovered there are many ways to do things, like loading the dishwasher. We all had to find creative ways to adjust prior-ities when an emergency came up. The best part of my first roommate experience was learning from each personality their cares and concerns. Roommates prepare you for marriage. Experiencing the rough grit of living with other people is a second tumbling—our first tumble is with family. I have noticed that living with family involves either a grace or a strictness that may keep you in the same habits and routine. When you change your environment, you learn more. It's like getting in a new barrel with new grit. Some of the rough edges that didn't get touched will find the grit to shape you.

I hope you find patient, kind roommates like I had. The first month, I partnered up with one of my roommates to do the cooking. We went grocery shopping together and bought all our food for the week. We added in a dozen muffins as a treat. Each day, the muffins were disappearing. I thought she was eating her share quickly, and she thought I was eating my share quickly. Later, we found out one of the other roommates was eating our food. Another time, I had a roommate who kept buying cars that broke down. She would get a cheap car, and it would break down, and she would have to get another cheap car, and it broke down. By her third car, the other cars were gathering dirt in the gutter from the parked cars in the street. The buildup in the ditch was causing a strong sewer smell. Finally, we gave her a month to get rid of the cars, or she had to move out and take the cars with her. She ended up moving out. Some of the personalities in the house were dancers, introverts, philosophers, trendy, sloppy, and hardly-ever-there roommates. There are so many stories we can look back on as roommates and laugh, cry, and be grateful for. Many times, we had each other to go on double or triple dates, have parties, or just hang out with. It was great to learn from each other and find a connection. The reason we got along for the most part, I believe, was that we had similar standards, and we agreed on rules. We all desired to be Christ focused as we pursued our educational and career goals.

If you plan to live with extended family, make sure you know what is expected of you. It will help if you write it out. List what you will pay and the areas of the home you are responsible for taking care of, and let them know your goal on staying there. Remember to give more than you take, even if it is just to take the trash out when you are not asked or do the dishes when you did not dirty them. Always add a bit more when you can to show your appreciation. If they do not ask anything from you, then it is even more important to take on some responsibility so you are growing.

Another option for moving out if you are the responsible type and have a job that pays you well enough, is to buy a home, townhome, or condo. Then you can find roommates to help you pay the mortgage. In order to buy a home, you will need to have a job that gives you an annual salary or a business that has been ongoing for more than two years, shows a profit, and pays you enough to qualify for a mortgage. It doesn't cost you anything to get professional advice from a real estate agent and a lender. You can talk to your bank or credit union, but I would suggest getting multiple opinions, including one from a mortgage broker. Mortgage brokers can shop around to different lending institutions to find the best deal for your situation. Buying a home or townhome can set you up for investing with the help of others to pay the debt while you enjoy income for years to come.

If home life is amazing and you get the opportunity to stay at home and not have to pay rent, then take on more responsibility to yourself. Set your goals, and make them big to set you up later when you do move out. How do you do this?

Budgeting.

Living at Home	Living on Your Own
50% Save	50% Bills
10% Give	10% Give
20% Bills	10% Save
20% Wants-Fun	20% Extra Expenses
	10% Wants-Fun

Let's talk about how to budget. When living at home, save 50 percent of your income. Ten percent will be for giving, whether it is your tithing or a cause you believe in. Make the habit of giving part of your life. I have found when I remember to give, I feel rich. I actually feel blessed and do better earning more. Twenty percent for bills. If you can discipline yourself to live on 20 percent of what you make, you will do well. The last 20 percent will be for fun, dates, entertainment, food, clothes, et cetera. If you don't have enough money to cover all that, either find some side hustles, sell items, get another job, or cut back on discretionary expenses—your "wants," like eating out and buying new clothes.

The more you can save, the more prepared you will be for emergencies. You may be saving for a big goal like a car, school, or a home, but there will always be an emergency that comes up, like the car battery dying or a tooth getting chipped. Be prepared if possible.

Once you move out, you will have more, larger expenses. This will cause the budget percentages to change. Typically, 50 percent ends up going to bills such as rent/mortgage, car payments, insurance, credit cards (try to avoid these, except one bank card to build credit, and pay it off each month), and cell phone. (You don't need the latest and greatest each year.) There are other monthly expenses like utilities, food, and gas that are variable and will take up 20 percent. Remember: 10 percent for giving and at least 10 percent for savings. That will leave the budget with 10 percent for fun and personal items.

Dave Ramsey is a money expert who helps people get out of debt. He has a budget graph that is a little different and another resource that I recommend. Keith and I used his snowball approach to paying off debt, which helped us get rid of three of Keith's student loans and a credit card balance.

	Amount Owed	Monthly Payment	Interest Rate	Payoff Goal
Mortgage	$100,000	$1,200	8%	
Student Loan 1	$6,500	$100	4%	
Student Loan 2	$3,200	$50	4%	Nov-Keith
Student Loan 3	$1,700	$25	4%	July 4-Keith
Car	$14,000	$250	5%	
Car	$7,800	$148	5%	
Credit Card	$3,700	$52	14%	Dec 8-Malissa
Box Store Credit	$1,200	$35	24.9%	Feb 26-Keith
Hospital	$600	$50	6%	March 1-Malissa

We made it a game. We listed all our creditors, the interest rates for each debt, how much we owed, and the monthly payment amounts in a spreadsheet. We posted it on the fridge. We each took a bill and added a date when we could pay it off. It was a race to see who could pay the one they selected off first. Then we took the money we would have paid on that bill and added it to the next one. We were now paying extra on the new bill, and that bill was paid off more quickly, and it just snowballed from there. We got really creative and sold anything we were not using, created a free-date-night list, and cooked at home.

I have found the easiest category to save on is the food budget. When I go to the grocery store hungry, I buy more food, and it tends to be the expensive, processed quick foods. That eats up my budget really quickly. The more I can cook from scratch, the better for my health and my pocketbook. When I can control my food budget, I can reach my money-saving goals quicker.

All these percentages plus Dave Ramsey's debt payoff method may feel like a lot right now. If it does, make this fun. The easiest way to get comfortable with a budget is to use fake money. I'll explain. When I was teaching in middle school, we had an activity once a year when professionals would come in to help with a simulation of the real world. To help the students understand some of the costs involved in living life, we gave them each a random scenario. They were single or married. Some had kids, and others were going to school. They went around to different tables that had an insurance provider, a banker, an auto dealer/ mechanic, a real estate agent, an accountant, a grocery store clerk, university staff, and a few other volunteers. As the students went around the room to find out how much things cost, they had to keep a tally on a life card. Then, in the process, each got a chance card, where they were hit with an unexpected life event and found out if they had an accident, had a child, or had to pay taxes. The students had to add that in and make adjustments. During many of the trips around the tables, they had choices of what car they would buy, where they would live, and whether they would go on a vacation. They were also given jobs randomly, so their income was determined by their jobs. Then they could choose to get an education to increase their pay.

It was a fun game, and it helped them discover some of the expenses in life and what careers they wanted to work toward. It helped them discover what educational route would be best for them, and then we discussed a plan for school and jobs to get them experience. Middle school is a nonthreatening time to explore and find out what you like. But even if you are out of high school, you can still explore. Many people in their forties are discovering better paths for themselves. Life is not a race; it is a time to learn and grow and shape yourself. You have to leave the nest someday, and I hope my experience can help you make a plan to get out on your own.

Wherever you're at right now, start there. Prepare for the future. Save as much money as you can now so that when you do move out (or to a bigger, nicer place), you'll be ready. Write down your goal for when you want to be out. Set a plan to save and increase your income to account for the increase of expenses.

Most people do not realize the cost of moving out until they are in the middle of the process and keep getting hit with more and more expenses. There are things to consider that you will have to pay besides rent. There will be utilities such as electricity, water, sewer, garbage, and internet. You will also need to have renter's insurance to cover your belongings if there is a disaster or a break-in, and things are stolen or destroyed. A good rule of thumb is that you should be earning three times your rent. So if the place you want to move into costs $1,000 a month, then you should be making $3,000 to live out on your own. But I have found many have done it for less. We did.

Other costs of moving out include all the small and big items you need in your new place, like dishes, silverware, a bed, a table and chairs, a couch, toilet paper, food, ketchup, mustard and maybe a washer and dryer. These things add up quickly and will take a major part of your budget.

If you can, collect those essentials now. When I was younger, I was given a hope chest. This was a big wooden chest like a trunk where I would put things I hoped to use when I got married or moved out on my own. I found some dishes I liked, bought them, and stored them in the chest. If you start to gather the smaller items, it will not cost as much when you move out. You can find good deals over time. Some places to find items at a great price are thrift and dollar stores. They have bowls, dishes, utensils, and many other good finds, sometimes for only a dollar. They are not the highest quality, but they're good enough to get by. I do recommend a good can opener, though. Nothing is as frustrating as not being able to open a can of food. Spend ten dollars on a good one. You will thank me later.

Other worthwhile investments for your first place are appliances. When I moved out and had to find a washer and a dryer, my budget was not high enough to buy new, so I had to find used ones. This was the time before Google, and finding items was not as easy as going to Facebook Marketplace, looking at the pictures, and messaging the seller. I had to look through the classifieds and call. I had to drive all over town to look at them, and I was not an expert, so I didn't even know if they were a good deal. I guessed and hoped and picked a set from a repairman that was within my budget. Then I had to figure out how to get them to the house. Luckily, I had a few friends with trucks. We got them, and then had to figure out how to hook them up. Growing up, I had never even looked behind the washer and dryer to see how they worked, and now I needed to hook them up. I had a friend smarter than me, and we got them running. The whole time I prayed that I had picked a good pair because this was all I had. I did get lucky. They lasted the whole time we rented that house.

I know I've thrown a lot of advice at you in this chapter. Because life throws a lot at you when you step out into the world as an adult, much of which you don't expect until it's right in front of you. One young couple I know, after putting a down payment on their first home, received a notice of foreclosure. The bank was going to kick them out because they hadn't paid the mortgage after three months. Apparently, they had no clue that when you "buy" a house, you don't actually *buy* the house. Nowadays, there is more education for first-time homeowners. I'm sure you know about mortgages and monthly payments, so I only bring up this story to point out how surprising the world can be to young people who are out on their own for the first time. It's my hope and prayer that what you learned from this chapter will make taking that step easier.

CHAPTER 7

Add More Grit: How to Get an Education without Going into Debt

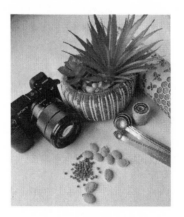

The things that we love tell us what we are.
—Saint Thomas Aquinas

By ninth grade, all my friends were talking about college. Most had older siblings who were planning to go the next year. We all talked about where we wanted to go. No one in my family had graduated from a university, so this was all new to me. I didn't know the first thing about going to college. My dad reminded me that I had free agency. If I wanted to do it, I would have to pay for it. He wanted me to take responsibility for my desires and invest in myself, so I figured out a way to get scholarships. It was a matter of self-respect. He reminded me never to tell myself I couldn't do something. Instead, he'd ask me, "How are you going to do that?" It's an empowering question rather than an enabling one. My dad reminded me that it was my decision and that I didn't have to go to college to get a good job or to create one.

My ninth-grade year really got me thinking and strategizing. I had to have a plan and build my resume. I joined as many clubs as I had time for. I played sports. I ran for student council. I saw an ad for a multischool newspaper that was looking for volunteers, so I offered to participate. I got involved with church activities. I had a part-time job. The scholarship committees wanted well-rounded individuals to give money to, so that is what I worked on over four years. How creative could I get? How could I stand out? Most importantly, what did I learn to love and hate by trying all these strategies?

Early in my senior year, I popped by the counseling office. Mrs. Hedge was in charge of the scholarships and would announce the ones that were available to apply for every morning. She became my advocate. Once she knew I was interested, she would send me notes in class about the current opportunities. One day, a new scholarship was announced all over the country—the Coca Cola Scholarship. They were offering $10,000 to thirty individuals for college. The application was a thick packet, but I was excited by the opportunity. That was a lot of money and could pay for all my schooling. I dreamed of how nice it would be not to have to work while going to school. I could go to my dream school where all my friends were going, BYU. I began the application process early and worked hard. Luckily, I had been involved in many activities that fit what they were looking for. I sent off my application. Months went by, and I made the finals. Wow, me, a finalist. Another packet. I was excited and started with the easy questions and requirements and put off the writing portion of the application. I had school, teams, and boys, which became a distraction. The deadline was approaching, but I stayed out late with a date instead of getting the writing done. When I got home to work on the final essay, I realized I had mixed up the dates. The application had to be postmarked by midnight on that day. I hurried and sealed it up, went to the post office late, and dropped it off. Not knowing how the post office worked at that age and living in Las Vegas, where everything is open twenty-four hours a day, I was hoping someone in the back of the post office would get my envelope and postmark it before midnight. My regrets were that I did not have someone proofread and edit it and that I procrastinated, which I hated. I was hoping for the good grace of the judges, but my application may have been kicked out before I even had a chance on the technicality of a postmark. As you probably guessed, I did not win the Coca Cola Scholarship, and I lost my dream school opportunity with all my friends. I did, however, win many small scholarships and a full-tuition scholarship to UNLV. A combination of all the little scholarships gave me enough for my first year of college and to help pay for room and board. I was accepted to BYU but got no scholarships. The decision was clear: I would be going to UNLV.

If you're in high school and you know what you want to do, set the plan, and get some experience to see if that is really what you want. A small part-time job, interning, or volunteering in the field that you are curious about can reveal quickly if this is the career for you. There are people who will help you if you are willing to give something a try and find your path. Many people want you to succeed.

Education is important, whether it is a formal education, a trade, or a skill. As long as you don't go broke for the rest of your life. I'm talking about those high-interest student loans that follow you forever. Student loans are the worst. Few things in this life or the next do I fear more than student loans. An entire generation of families is not being formed because their would-be parents can't even afford to buy a house and get married, much less provide for a child while Mama stays home. Student loan payments are devouring the budget.

Please, for the sake of your future husband, children, and children's children, *do not finance your education.* You deserve better than lifelong bondage, and there are many ways to raise the funds. Only a few degrees deserve student loans—typically, a medical, legal, or other high-earning professional degree—but even then, the military will help with the funding. All I am saying is to be very cautious when you accept a student loan. It may seem like easy money, but paying it back is a big burden for most.

Do you want to pursue one of those highly intense professions when you grow up? You don't have to if you don't want to, and that's OK. Many people don't know what they are going to college for. They are still discovering. Why not get paid to find out? Then, if college is the answer, go further with your dream of becoming the best at what you want to be. Why not?

The point again is do not get into debt to pursue a career you may not even enjoy—or make any money at. Working with the resources you have, which may be less money, helps you live with just the essentials and be creative on how to get by. This is where true growth can occur. If you have time to prepare, start early with the system that is in place to earn scholarships and grants.

And while you're getting your education, don't spend money you don't have. Multigenerational living is OK. There is nothing wrong with living at home to save money. Just don't freeload. Make sure to add value and keep your relationships intact. You may have to stay within the family rules, assist with household chores, and be respectful, but nothing is wrong with that. We always told our kids that if they were going to school, they had the option of living with us without rent. They were still expected to pull some weight and keep up responsibilities at home. We did not want to encourage irresponsible adults, and staying at home is a privilege, not a right. It was our way to help them so they did not have to take out student loans. Don't deny yourself the chance to create great stories of struggle as you get an education. I had a room-mate who didn't tell us she was broke and ate potatoes for a month because that was all she could afford. You can get creative for dates and make a list of all the free things to do in your town.

This is good both when you're single and when you're married. I remember when my kids were young, we would get a video from the library, which was free; make popcorn; and have a night in. The kids got to be in their pj's, and we enjoyed the comfort of home. Through hard times, many have learned to enjoy their homes more. We just have to be creative. Outdoor activities can be free: try going to a park, creating a treasure hunt or photo hunt around town, taking a walk and talking, or making everyday tasks fun, which my son did when he went grocery shopping with a date. He was blindfolded, and she had to direct him to the items on the list.

Learning to cook and eating at home can save money and is healthier than going out to eat all the time. Have a contest and see what you can add to make the best bowl of ramen. Get cookie-cutters and make your food into fun shapes—kids love them and so do adults. You may also enjoy mashing up international dishes, like Tex-Mex tacos with Asian chili spices or bowls of Vietnamese phở soup with Italian pasta instead of rice noodles. There are so many ideas; maybe that will be my next book, or I'll list them on the website, www.lifetumbled.com. What I'm saying is enjoy the struggle. It is your time to grind the jagged edges, and I want you to know your options and put the best tools in your tool belt for life. Take on the challenge so you can go for your dreams.

Everyone dreams of a stable, secure career. However, times have changed. Where we work is different now—there's the office, the home office, the cafes with Wi-Fi, and mobile hotspots that bring internet access to wherever you are. Career advice that worked for most people even ten years ago won't work for most of us in this new world. That said, the one stable career path that has survived and even thrived during technological and social change has been learning a trade. Technical careers promise higher-paying jobs with less (and less expensive) schooling needed to build them. Career and technical opportunities, what the education industry calls CTE, focus more on skill than theory. Naturally, they prioritize actual experience over books and classrooms. CTE career paths include:

- Health sciences
- Business
- Marketing and sales
- Finance
- Information technology
- STEM
- Manufacturing
- Logistics
- Hospitality

- Government
- Public safety
- Agriculture
- Human services
- Construction
- Training
- Arts

Some CTE career paths require a university degree, others a trade degree or certificate. All require experience, which you get in the field right away. The more experience you have, the better your chance of figuring out if you like it, getting a job you love, and having the option to work for someone else or be an entrepreneur. The best news is that because these professions are in high demand, many employers are willing to foot the bill for your formal education *and* pay you to learn on the job. That's a deal.

Jump in wherever you can in a field you might be interested in. You can volunteer, job shadow, and network within the community to create experiences that help you find what you love, pad your resume, and build your savings.

Don't know how to find what you like and what direction you want to go in? Try to remember what you liked to do as a kid. Also, make a list of all the things you hate to do. The fastest way to find something you like is to cut out what you don't like. Look for jobs online and see what descriptions sound interesting or fun or pique your curiosity. Once you find a job description that seems interesting, look at the qualifications they ask for and start by gaining those skills.

Here's a constructive activity that will help you. Create a spreadsheet with two columns. In column one, write the skills and experience you can prove you have on your resume. In column two, write the skills and experience you need for your ideal job or the next job you want. Then fill in the gaps by volunteering, interning, job shadowing, or anything else you can think of to develop and gain experience in those areas.

When I lived in the small town of Sterling, there was not much to do, and I did miss the big-city events. I have always had a desire to gather the community together and help small businesses. My mother-in-law worked for the American Cancer Society and put on events all over the state of Utah. She needed some help to start the Sanpete County Relay for Life, which is a twenty-four-hour relay to raise money for cancer study and patients in need. I told her I would help her put the event together. She introduced me to many people in the county: representatives and business owners. We got the students at the college involved and held the event on campus. We worked on it for months and developed some great relationships. The community really came together, and we were able to raise $6,000 in a low-income county. This was an amazing amount for the community and my first fundraiser at the young age of twenty-one. Everything I'd learned from high school activities such as art club, honor society, and student council came together to make the event a success.

Many people in the community saw my work ethic and how well I was able to work with others. Actually, that is how I landed a job at the college while I finished my degree. It also gave me the opportunity to put together the first bridal fair for the county. The Manti Temple is located in Sanpete County, and it is a destination wedding location. This is what most of the bed-and-breakfast houses survive on. The economic developer saw an opportunity to help the businesses in the county and recruited me to pull the event together. One thing led to another—all from volunteering to help with the Relay for Life event.

When I moved from Sterling to Tooele, I started the Relay for Life in that county and then was asked to speak at the Tooele Small Business Conference to help women with work. Working at Snow College gave me experience in education and event planning. The successful Relay for Life events led to the job at the University of Utah, and it goes on and on. All this and more just for dumping my "nevers" (remember, I was never going to live in Utah, live in a small town, or work for family), jumping in, and helping my mother-in-law with her bed-and-breakfast.

As you pursue career opportunities, expand yourself as a person with a well-rounded temporal and spiritual education. Decide who you want to be and what that might look like—for example: a confident, industrious, and faithful individual. Understand that you become what you do. Attend seminary, institute, church, youth conference, and girls' camp. Dive deep into the scriptures. You will find yourself naturally manifesting the fruit of the spirit in your life in all areas. Where before you may have struggled with fear or grudges, you will have only love for yourself and others. Where there was inner turmoil, you will have joy and peace. A short temper will be no more, replaced by patience, kindness, and goodness. Procrastination out, faithfulness in. And others will be drawn to your newfound gentleness, meekness, and self-control. This will all feel perfectly normal. You won't have to pretend to be someone you are not because you *will be* this person.

I have found that spiritual growth keeps me grounded in what is really important. The distractions of the world can carry us away and make us forget the real journey of eternal life. Many times, the scripture stories have helped me. By going to seminary, I found my favorite scripture pops into my mind whenever I'm worried life might be taking a wrong turn.

> Search diligently, pray always, and be believing, and all things shall work together for your good, if ye walk uprightly and remember the covenant wherewith ye have covenanted one with another.
> —Doctrine and Covenants 90:24, Book of Mormon

This verse specifically—and scripture reading generally—have helped me through really tough times. As a family, we barely survived the 2007–2008 economic downturn. Keith lost his job, and we had to move (all five of us) into my mother's house. She had just moved into my stepdad's condo to care for him during cancer treatment, and she needed me to help care for my special-needs sister.

In the midst of these financial and personal crises, I could still find blessings. My older sister would remind me to "be like the lilies"—the Lord knows what we need even before we ask. He will provide. Have faith and keep moving forward. It's up to us to thoughtfully and prayerfully invest the resources we have. Remember those who have gone before us and the sacrifices they have made to allow us to be where we are today. And remember . . . someone always has it worse than you, and many still find joy.

Eventually, the economy restarted. So did our lives. We got through. If I hadn't had fasting, prayer, scriptures, and family gospel discussions to comfort me when I felt weak, I might not have recovered from my own depression and anxiety as the rest of the world recovered from the economic recession.

Making a living will get you far in good times and bad. But only grounding your life in the truth of God's Word will help you outlast any trial, tribulation, or temptation.

CHAPTER 8

Get a Bigger Barrel: How to Make Money without Making Yourself Crazy

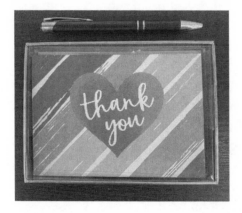

It's pretty hard for the Lord to guide you if you haven't made up your mind which way to go.
—Madam C. J. Walker

Most people know two ways to earn money. You either work for someone else as an employee, or you create your own job as an entrepreneur. The choice is yours. Each has pros and cons.

My degree is in education. Nobody gets into that field for the money. My husband was also in education, and we both had to have side jobs to make ends meet. Keith worked construction. I could always find a business idea, but most of the time, I was afraid to move forward out of a fear of failure or of what people might think. Whenever I focused on myself—*I* needed this to work—it held me back. When I could see how my ideas could help others, they worked. One of my businesses was photography, which made me nervous at first. So many fears ran through my mind, but I kept working at it and got better and better. When you work on mastering a skill, opportunities will come your way. It all comes down to what you are more afraid of: starving or what people think. OK, maybe you are not at that point, and you just want some extra cash. Let's get your juices flowing.

My first job working for someone else (besides opening a lemonade stand and babysitting) came at the age of twelve. I saw an ad in a magazine for people to sell stationery and paper products door to door. This opportunity allowed me to earn my own money and win my own stationery. I can still remember the smell of the new, fresh paper in its own box. I couldn't wait to write a letter to my grandmother. In middle school and high school, I sold candy. My dad taught us how to buy the candy and sell it for a profit and then take the money and buy more to grow the business. That set me up for other small businesses. One summer, I bought glow sticks and had my brother and kids help me sell them at the fair. In two hours, I could pay my brother twenty dollars and have enough for groceries for the month.

Nowadays, there are so many opportunities, including the internet. Nothing should stop you. (Unless it's illegal or sinful!) My niece's four-year-old daughter set up a pop shop (new-age lemonade stand) outside her home during a busy Parade of Homes event and made $150 in three hours. She is adorable and persuasive. Her parents built the stand and helped her chill and set up the soda pop, but she made it happen. She was not afraid to ask people to buy her lemonade.

Fear is what holds us back from selling ourselves. Every time I think of a business idea that didn't work out or that I didn't even try, the culprit was fear. I felt afraid of what people might think when they saw me promoting it. What if I didn't succeed? The question ought to have been "What if I *do* succeed?" What if this is amazing? I have special gifts and desires, and so do you. Don't be afraid to let your light shine, whether that means selling to family and friends, to neighbors, or to the world over the internet.

If you don't attend college for a four-year degree, that's not to say your only viable alternative is sales—either selling your own product or service or promoting someone else's through a commissioned sales job. Remember Chapter 6 and the CTE? The skilled trades are an option for everyone, especially for young women.

Many girls think they will grow up and get married and not need an education. I'm here to tell you that 100 percent of females need to have a skill or an education. It doesn't have to be a formal education. And not necessarily for a particular job. The biggest reason is to shape our individuality. Our purpose on earth is to learn and grow, and sometimes we will need to rely on the education we sought.

My mom's dad died when she was eight, and my grandmother had to go to work. My dad died, and my mom had to go to work. My sister was divorced, and she had to go to work. My husband was sick, and I had to go to work. We can choose to work outside the home or create a side hustle. Nowadays, more people work from home than ever before, and that is a great opportunity and a blessing for those who are better at supporting another's dream and helping him or her succeed. We all have our abilities and passions. It's better to be the best number two (or twenty-two) on the corporate ladder than to be an entrepreneur and not make ends meet. Find what makes you happy and be the best version of yourself. Always be learning and getting better. You're only competing with yourself.

I am the first to admit it doesn't always feel that way. What makes us crazy is observing other people and wanting what they have. I have found that envy or coveting another's life will stop a person in their path. They may see what they think is the perfect way of life on social media, but in reality, they do not know what is under the surface or the work it took to get there. There is no rule book or single path. My family has tried both nine-to-five and entrepreneurship. My dad was in construction and always believed a person could create their own job. My husband and I both worked in education until we went out on our own. My son worked in photography and videography for the Bureau of

Land Management until his business started to increase. My second son is a screen printer while working at Costco until he can get his business up and running out of our garage. We do what we can when we follow our heart.

The hard part for me is following my heart in only one direction at a time. It's difficult to pick one idea to dedicate time and energy to. When it comes to business ideas, job opportunities, and career paths, I'm like a girl in a candy store. Other people feel like castaways at sea—which direction is best for me? I want to try them all; you may have no idea what you want to do with your life or even what's possible. Find someone doing something you find fascinating and move in that direction. You may switch directions, and that is OK. Just don't give up too soon. It's the grind that creates our character.

In any case, implementation is the hard part. I can create and plan all day long, but at some point, I have to struggle through some rough points to keep the idea moving along. That's why you need to love something about your work. You may see the bigger picture of why it needs to happen so you can push through.

Because it takes a lot of effort to make any one idea work, I recommend several little tests—side hustles—to see which idea resonates and can generate revenue. How do you get started running these experiments? The way to find a side hustle is to see a need in an area that you like and offer a solution. You can also ask people close to you what you are good at, make a list, and go from there, investigating things you like and that bring joy. It's OK if you are scared—that means you are growing.

At one point, I thought I should start a preschool in my home. I had my education degree, but I didn't know if people would sign their kids up. I never went to preschool and didn't know the opportunities other families invested in with their children. There was a great need that I didn't comprehend at the time. I decided not to do it because of all the unknowns. I was afraid and couldn't see the opportunity, and I missed the experience of being at home with my family. But there are so many opportunities out there. Another door opened, and I ended up getting a job as an educational talent search adviser at the middle and high school, which grew my love for helping students find post-secondary education and scholarships and transition into adulthood. It was one of my best jobs.

While there are only two ways to earn money, you don't have to try one or the other or even only one at a time. Life itself is an experiment. We test; we measure; we figure out what to do next. No path is linear. Like me, you may get some college, try your hand at entrepreneurship, and pivot to traditional full-time employment, or you may not switch around and stick with one path. Ultimately, work adds value to your life and to the people around you.

I encourage you to be an industrious woman and create an interesting path in pursuit of joy.

CHAPTER 9

Clean Out the Barrel: How to Stay Healthy without Being a Health Nut

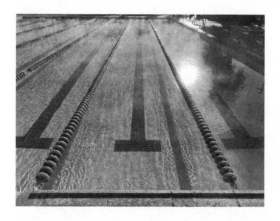

To keep the body in good health is a duty. Otherwise we shall not be able to keep our mind strong and clear.
—Gautama, the Lord Buddha

Have you seen the *I Love Lucy* episode where Lucy and Ethel are working in a candy factory? The conveyor belt is sending chocolates down the line, and Lucy and Ethel have to wrap them before they get to the shipping department. Our bodies are the same way. If we eat too much, we can't keep up. The body has to store all those excess calories somewhere, and that somewhere is fat all over our bodies.

The brain works similarly. We can be bombarded with demands from work, school, family, and social media. We can fill our schedules with overwhelming numbers of to-dos. If you don't set boundaries, anxiety can build up quickly. People with a helping nature can give their schedule away to others and lose their sense of self.

My mother encouraged all her kids to have hobbies and grow our talents. I loved art and played high school sports. These were great ways to relieve stress. When I got married, Keith and I ran together on date night. It was cheap, and it was therapy. Running helped me relax and think. I felt that runner's high even when my body was exhausted. This taught me that if anything went wrong or got stressful at work, I could go for a run and calm down.

In October 2019, a car accident took that away from me. A careless driver's mistake tore the tissue between my L4 and L5 vertebrae. The pinched nerve shot pain down my right leg. For a year and a half, I tried to find something to replace running, something that didn't bring agonizing pain or put me flat in bed. Friends suggested swimming and yoga. I don't like the water, especially in the winter, and the yoga classes were not at a convenient time. Excuses, I know. I liked running. I endured the grit to build that habit, and finally, it was comfortable. I hated trying to find something new. But what choice did I have? Sitting in an office chair all day isn't exactly relaxing or inspirational as a place to think. Finally, I admitted the truth—I had to look at another sharp edge and try to grind it to my benefit.

A year and a half after the accident, my son asked me to go swimming with him. It felt easy to say yes this time. I wanted to get away. People were on spring break, and I had to work. I figured I'd just take the weekend for a staycation. I did enjoy swimming and the spa when I was away, so why not spend more time at the gym than usual?

So there I was at the pool. My son started with his usual warm-up routine, and I waded in slowly. There was a slight warmth to the air, and the water was just right. I took a relaxing lap, not pushing myself. I just wanted to enjoy the moment. After several laps, my mind began to open like it did when I would run. Ideas came into my mind. My breathing slowed, and I really enjoyed myself. The guy in the lane next to me had a few interesting items to help with his swim. He had these web gloves on his hands. I asked him why, and he let me know they gave a better workout. That day, I decided to look into swimming a bit more. I did not have the pain I had from running, and it gave me a similar result. I realized it had been me in my way. I had not wanted to grind a new habit. My son asked if we could swim every morning. I happily agreed. I had found my new release.

• • • •

Health is a lifestyle. What you eat. What you think. What you do.

There is so much advice out there about exercising, eating, and taking care of yourself generally. Eat this; don't eat that. Do this; don't do that. And then, years later, it's OK to eat the same things they told you would kill you.

Here's my advice: do everything in moderation. Eat in moderation. Cut back on sugar. I have a dear friend who ate no sugar for a year without exercise and trimmed up, beautiful and healthy. I think we just need to be aware of what we are putting into our bodies. Will it help or hurt? Is this a craving for me and my taste buds, or will this help my body grow healthy?

I know it is easier said than done, especially with social media. You see the giant pile of ice cream drizzled with fudge and caramel that you and your favorite fifteen friends couldn't eat all together or that wacky donut or strange food that you have to try and keep trying and trying. I'm right there with you. I love trying new things. I love sharing with friends. I love to bake and cook. But sometimes even I don't have time for the kitchen, and I grab things because they're convenient.

With a little planning and conscientiousness, we can help our bodies function properly by feeding them what will help and not hurt. Sundays are always a good day to plan the week. I have a chalkboard on my wall on which I plan a weekly menu. I may not follow it to the letter, but it does give me ideas so I don't have to think. Some days, I will cook a different meal because I am in the mood for it that day. This also helps with grocery shopping. I can see what's in my pantry, cook with what I have, and make a list of the items that I need.

We ate at home most of the time when I was raising my family. We had a little game. I would make dinner. Everyone would rate it on a scale of one to ten, with ten being the best, and that would mean I should make it as often as I could. Also, I would have everyone guess how much it cost to feed the family that night. Many times, our family of five could eat for five or six dollars, and it tasted great. We all loved this challenge. It was our tradition. It also helped us when we went out to eat to decide if it was really worth it. When we made food at home, it was cheaper, and we'd have leftovers. It tasted better and was better for us.

We have always had a garden, which gave us fresh food. Nothing beats fresh onions or broccoli from the garden. Pick some spinach first thing in the morning for a smoothie or tomatoes, peppers, and cilantro for homemade salsa. Gardening can bring a healthy lifestyle into a home. Also, digging in the dirt with the sun hitting your skin can bring a sense of peace to one's life. It's a lot like running except the whole family can enjoy the fruits of your effort. And the vegetables.

Poor mental health—anxiety in particular—is a major problem today. It is something to be constantly vigilant about, and creating a habit to get you through the day should be a high priority. I'm not a therapist, but some of the solutions that have helped me are writing in my journal; spreading sunshine to someone else with service or dropping off something little; prayer; talking with a friend; writing a personal note; going for a walk outside; drawing; and, of course, exercising.

Personal notes have meant so much to me over the years that they deserve more than a brief mention. They're beneficial for the writer as well as the receiver. I love writing notes to people, maybe because I feel it is one way to really brighten someone's day. Many times, people don't really know what we think of them and how we may admire or appreciate the way they have influenced us. They could have given us something small as a smile or given generously at a special event. If you send a note in gratitude for that moment, it lifts you again and will lift the other person too.

I wrote one special note that changed a relationship for me when a friend was helping me with my business. We had been working together for years. Then I was introduced to someone who said they could do the job better, so I switched my business over to the new individual. Several months passed. The new individual made some major mistakes, and I knew I had made a bigger one. I humbly asked my friend to take over. I wrote her a note to let her know what I admired in her. I wondered what she would think and whether this would be awkward, but I sent the note anyway. That note is what bound us to a stronger friendship.

I can actually tell you many stories of how a note changed someone's life. There was a woman who wrote five notes a day because she had the same joy in writing personal notes. Later in her life, when she wanted to run for mayor, she won in a landslide. Months before his passing, my father wrote me a note and left it in my car; I hold that note dear and can reread it to give me strength during hard times. My relationship with my husband grows closer every time he writes me a note. It's always a good feeling to be reminded of the good people see in you. Do you like personal notes too?

While you care for your mental and emotional health and that of those you love, remember you are an eternal being. I have found that strong spiritual health will get you through the roughest times. First, understand your Heavenly Father loves you and wants what's best for you. Find answers in the scriptures. Many times, when I have a question on my mind, I'll study it, pray, and then get my answer when reading the stories in the scriptures. Those were people who lived. They had struggles and thoughts. Through their faith and diligence, they found the answers. Some answers are harder to act on than others, but if we remember to act with the motive of doing what is best from an eternal perspective and not what we want right now, sometimes, the answers are easy and fun.

Many times in our lives, we pray for answers, and the Lord will guide us, and other times, He allows us to make the decision. He is not always going to tell us what to do. Sometimes there are two right decisions, and it is your choice. Look at the brother of Jared in the Book of Mormon. The Lord gave him the task of building some boats and told him how to construct them. There was one problem. They were built so tight that neither air nor light could get in. The brother of Jared prayed for answers. The Lord told him how to add two holes for air but gave him the task of finding a way to let in light. The brother of Jared found stones and asked the Lord to touch the stones so they would light up, and they could use them on their journey. Sometimes there is no one right answer; there are many ways. We can get caught up in the assumption that we have to hear the answer directly from God. And if we don't, we will do the wrong thing. Many choices are between two right options. Just pick one. This simple fact will do wonders for your spiritual growth as well as your emotional well-being and mental health.

Ultimately, optimal health in every area of life becomes a lifestyle. There was a study done by researchers who called five regions in the world Blue Zones. They all had similar lifestyles, and they had the most centurions (individuals who lived more than one hundred years) in the world. The people who live the longest typically take care of their bodies, minds, *and* spirits. They move their bodies every day and eat greens and whole foods. They have a social support group that encourages them in healthy ways. They take time to relax and destress. They are part of a community that is religious and in which they serve. They are also committed to their families and have a sense of purpose.

That all sounds great in theory, but what about in real life? Nurturing your physical, mental, and spiritual health simultaneously is not as complex as it sounds. Like we learned in goal setting, accomplishing one meta goal can make several dreams come true. I found that in the Body for Life Challenge.

After having my last baby, I gained the most weight and was the sickest. It was hard to lose the weight. I tried on my own during what was the hardest year of my life. My father had been tragically killed, and I sank into a deep depression to the point that scriptures and prayer didn't feel like they did anything anymore.

Then I had a spontaneous conversation with my brother. He said he wanted to get back into shape. I did too.

"Want to do the Body for Life Challenge?" he asked.

"What's that?"

Body for Life is a twelve-week nutrition and exercise program with an annual physique transformation competition. They award $100,000 to the person or group with the most improvement. We'd have to take before and after photos. For additional motivation and support, there is a book and website to help with meals and workouts. They provide a schedule of workouts: upper body Monday, twenty minutes of cardio Tuesday, legs Wednesday, twenty minutes of cardio Thursday, upper body Friday, and cardio on Saturday. Sunday was a day of rest. A body needs to rest. And then the next week, you pick up with legs on Monday. It looked simple on paper.

Eating seemed like it would be simple too. Eat a serving of protein, vegetables, and whole grains, each the size of your palm. No sugar except Sunday, which is your cheat day. Even though it seemed simple, it was a challenge. Financially, could I afford to go to a gym? Luckily, my brother had a connection to a gym. Check. Would I have the money to buy nutritional food? My food budget was balanced because I didn't buy processed foods. What if I got injured and had to have down days? I worked through all of them day by day and was patient with myself. Sometimes just starting and being persistent is all you need.

It helped to have my brother as a partner. He held me accountable; I didn't want to be the weak link in this competition. We got up at 5:00 a.m. to go to the gym. We had to get up early because we both had jobs, and we had to squeeze in time to accomplish this goal. Time was the major hurdle to overcome. We had to create a new routine and still have energy throughout the day. It took some time to adjust, and knowing I had someone waiting for me helped.

Amazingly, after the Body for Life Challenge, I was able to run a part of the 2002 Salt Lake City Winter Olympic Torch Relay. I nominated my husband through the Chevrolet sponsorship, and in return, the relay committee asked me to run too. It was an exciting opportunity. We ran the first day the torch was in Utah. I ran in the center of downtown, and Keith got the opportunity to hand the torch off to the final runner before it stopped for the evening. A very memorable moment: I was on the shuttle being transported to my leg of the run. As we dropped each person off at their spot, there were crowds of people cheering and shaking the shuttle. I felt like a superstar and received a ton of energy from the crowd. I really felt like I could do anything. The positive energy filled us up.

Before we got on the shuttle, we were given instructions on how to accept the eternal flame. It was propane powered, and there was an assistant who would turn on our torch before we accepted the flame. As the runner approached, I angled my torch to catch the flame of theirs. I did not want this moment to end, so I started off slow and then began to run. I heard my brother say, "Malissa, you can run faster than that!"

Several months later, I got to be the last leg of the relay for the Special Olympics. I was truly blessed to have had this opportunity. The theme for the Olympics was Light the Fire Within. I had been a common girl who now felt extraordinary. My thoughts about myself changed, so it felt like *I* changed. Never underestimate the power of the mind.

When Muhammed Ali trained to be the best boxer in the world, he did not count his reps until they began to hurt. His reasoning was that the mind will have you quit before you've accomplished all you really can. Your mind will put limits on you and create a reality that is less than your potential. Your mind is so powerful. A mantra I often tell myself is "Think good thoughts, and you will do good deeds." When I have trouble getting my thoughts in order, I exercise or go for a walk. At the same time, I put on good music or listen to a podcast or book that can train my mind to go down the path of productive thinking instead of tearing myself down or allowing Satan to manipulate my thinking. Whenever we start to feel jealous, covetous, or sorry for ourselves, that is a sure sign that we should get our minds into the gym of good thoughts. It takes training, and it's a constant exercise to keep your thoughts clean and uplifting. Just like eating is a way of life, so are your thoughts, and your thoughts are the beginning of making you great.

During the Body for Life Challenge, my mental capacities were strengthened when I reached my goal of lifting a certain weight. I started out gradually. We did sets of twelve, ten, eight, and six. The weight on the rep of six was to be as heavy as I could do and still keep proper form. I made it my goal to add more weight on each rep on Monday and have that new weight amount feeling easy to lift by Saturday. The gradual progress was hard to see, but tracking and keeping records opened my eyes to what I could do. I gave myself small challenges each week and by the time the twelve weeks were complete, I had improved more than I thought possible.

As an individual, I was happier. This new exercise routine was giving me endorphins, and I could handle some stresses that used to cripple me. It gave me a brighter outlook, which people started to notice. Early morning was my quiet time to breathe and have peace with my mind. It was time for me. Nowadays, I can turn on scriptures and podcasts to tune in to the spirit. The "read your scriptures daily" routine became a bit easier. I don't always listen to scriptures, but on the days I need the Lord the most, I certainly do.

The Lord wants you to live a joyous life. Keep your mind, body, and spirit healthy. You can choose to be happy.

An exercise that has helped with my mental survival is writing in my journal. I use this as a way to rid myself of frustrations and say what I really want to say. It helps me flush out my feelings. Writing things out on paper helps me release them from my subconscious, which may want to hold on to them and burst when I have had enough. Sometimes I burn or shred journal entries if what I have to say is pulling me down and making me angry. I could hurt someone I care about with the words I write when I'm emotional. I have learned from others never to post on social media when I am angry or feeling emotional. Never. In fact, I have given myself a break from social media. Take a break and cleanse your thoughts from the bombardment of social stimulus.

I have a dear friend from high school, Terresa, who writes in her journal every day. She is one to admire with a shelf full of journals. She loves to write. The power of journaling can bring more happiness, help you attain your goals, and keep you healthy. I have learned to write in my journal when I want to pray for others as a way to remember the blessings and answers to prayers that have come my way. And, most importantly, to write down what I am grateful for.

A popular and effective journaling technique is keeping a gratitude journal. My mind tends to go to negative thoughts, and when I can write what I'm grateful for each morning, it sets me off to a good start. A gratitude journal may be a struggle to start, but as soon as I became consistent, it trained my brain to be more joyful. A gratitude journal can remind you of the good times. Help boost you when you're down. Remind yourself of the things you have accomplished. And, most importantly, help you rest your mind. Put any and all racing thoughts onto paper. That includes writing notes to people and sending them in the mail. It's like a mini Sabbath for your brain.

Just like the spirit needs a day of rest from this temporal existence, our bodies do too. Fasting is the opportunity to give your body the needed rest and the ability to clean out toxins. If you are a member of the Church of Jesus Christ of Latter-day Saints, you are familiar with the practice of fasting once a month for twenty-four hours or two meals. You may have been brought up to do this as a tradition to bring you closer to God spiritually and to find answers. I certainly was. I have a testimony on the power of fasting for spiritual benefits. It has been in my later years that I have discovered the health benefits too. It is amazing how the Lord gives us words of wisdom that help us in multiple ways.

Over these past ten years, as I have studied the effects of fasting on my body, I have learned that most times, it clears my mind and gives me energy. When we eat too much, the body takes energy to process the food. That's why after gorging at Thanksgiving, we want to take a nap. Our body is working overtime to get the food through our system.

During this time of rest and fasting, the body is able to clean out and rejuvenate, like spring cleaning. Autophagy is the process by which the cells in our bodies clean up, like taking out the trash. At night when we sleep, our bodies are working to clean up. If we eat a late-night snack, our bodies can't clean up because they have to process what is coming through our system. If we choose to stop eating around six or seven and let our bodies work through the night while fasting, we will be able to maintain a healthy lifestyle. Studies show that fasting can reduce inflammation, improve overall health, and sharpen the mind. Many times, when we think we are hungry, we are actually thirsty. Drink some water before going to the fridge for a snack.

Always consult your doctor before you start any new regime of exercise and diet changes. But remember to talk to the Great Physician about them first.

CHAPTER 10

Tumble Together: How to Pick a Good One

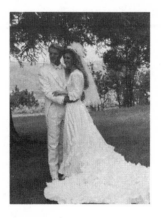

I can conquer the world with one hand, as long as you are holding
the other.
—Unknown

In high school, my friend Tammy liked a certain boy. She wasn't in
the habit of showing interest in a boy, any boy, most of the time, but
she focused on one particular boy, Ryan. She would go to the wrestling
matches to watch him; hang out with him; and buy him clothes, smooth-
ies, and snacks. They were never boyfriend/girlfriend, but they hung out
a lot of the time. She wanted more, but Ryan liked to date around. He
broke her heart many times. He didn't treat her with respect and probably knew she would always be around. When high school was complete,

Ryan went on a mission. They wrote to each other. Tammy was the support, always lifting him up.

Six months before Ryan was to finish his mission, a friend of Tammy's set her up on a date with Trevor. The three of them were going golfing. Trevor had had a crush on Tammy in high school but was too shy to ask her out. Tammy had been so focused on Ryan that she'd hardly noticed Trevor except that he was cute and always kind to her. Trevor was popular and on the student council. Tammy didn't think she would even have a chance with him.

The mission wasn't for Ryan, and he ended up coming home early. He tried to reconnect with Tammy and pull her in with his emotional needs. Tammy was always there, but she was really enjoying her time with Trevor. It wasn't long before Trevor asked Tammy to be his girlfriend, and Tammy loved being around him. Ryan began to get clingy and told Tammy that he had prayed and knew Tammy was the one for him. Tammy was confused. How could that be? Was she supposed to be with Ryan? All these years she had wanted to be with him, but who was the right one for her?

Tammy and I had an institute class together called Marriage Preparation. I remember the class so clearly. The instructor told us that marriage was the most important decision we would ever make. The way he said it stuck with me and hit Tammy the same way. After class, we discussed her situation. She could see Ryan was not good for her, but she was emotionally connected, and Ryan had prayed and gotten an answer. I told her that she needed to pray and fast for her answer and to list the pros and cons of both Ryan and Trevor. I could see that Ryan was not the one, and Trevor was the better choice, but she had to come to the conclusion. I could see that her life would be different with each one just by the way she carried herself and her outlook on life when she was in their presence. I felt that I could see her with more joy if she chose Trevor, but she had to make the decision. I did not want her to pick Ryan out of guilt.

Luckily, she did her own praying, fasting, and pondering in her heart and did pick Trevor. They ended up getting married and are so cute together.

Now to the real stuff. Just because they are cute together does not mean everything is perfect. Marriage is a quick way to find out people do things differently. Differences matter, but they don't. Disagreements on the little things, like how to arrange dishes and silverware or the "right" way to prepare macaroni and cheese, are opportunities to work together to find an agreeable solution. Marrying someone who is reasonable in disagreements matters so much more than marrying someone you agree with about every single thing.

If I had a magic wand and could create the perfect guy for you, this is what I would create: a young man who will be your friend with integrity, loyalty, patience, hard work, kindness, laughter, health, intelligence, and confidence. A continual learner and service oriented. Most importantly, he loves the Lord. He will be spiritually grounded and have an abundant mindset. In order to find someone like that, you must be working on yourself, and you may not find a one-and-done guy like this. We are all works in progress, and it is what's in our hearts that is most important. Learn to recognize motives and mindsets.

Let's talk about the motive in someone's heart and the mindset of whether or not they think they can do something. Being able to understand someone's heart and why they do something will help you understand what motivates them and why they do it. Is it out of love? Fear? Ego?

Motives are the reasons someone does something. Many people are unconscious of their own motives, let alone anyone else's. The sooner you can discern people's motives, the sooner you will gain your emotional intelligence. This will give you strength, and you will be able to respond appropriately. The less people can manipulate your emotions, the more control you have over your future.

How do you find out someone's motives? I have found it can take days, weeks, or months. First, look at their actions. How do they conduct themselves? How do they treat others who can't give anything in return, and how do they treat people who don't have a strong voice or opinion? A second sign is a person's speech. Are they fast talkers and just say what you want to hear? Do they play on your emotions? The third way to discover a person's motive is to have a discussion with them. Let them talk about their dreams, their inner desires, their true motives, and what drives them.

What are the motives of the person who wants to marry you? Do they care about your well-being, or do they want to control you? Do they let you explore your desires, or do they want someone to take care of them? What are their insecurities that pull you in or repel you?

A couple of times while I was dating, I caught a glimpse of a motive that made me uncomfortable, and I soon realized why this person was dating me. Some guys wanted to control me. As soon as I felt that motive, that was the end of spending time with them. Others were open and wanted to have fun. They wanted to discover what I enjoyed and what I loved about life. They protected my individuality. Some even amplified it with encouragement. One clue to a person's motives is whether they take your agency away. Do they let you make choices? Do your motives match?

In the same way you vet potential mates, vet yourself. By that I mean, allow yourself the self-awareness to realize how you may become more attractive. I'm not talking about physical appearance. I mean how you approach life itself. Over the years, I've studied the victim-and-player mentalies. Are you the *victim* or a *player* in life?

A victim is someone who lets life hit them, and then they dwell on that situation and may even blow it up to create more drama. The victim mentality makes a person resistant to correction. This type of thought process will attract personalities and create an environment of nonprogression. In dating it will attract the controlling and manipulating individuals and repel the people who see life full of opportunity.

Sometimes the victim mentality is actually trying to control the other person by drawing them in to get the other person's help. That is how they keep them in the relationship. Ryan was trying to keep my friend Tammy with his victim mentality, and when that didn't work and Tammy saw a different way to live, Ryan created a gaslighting situation. He was psychologically manipulating her to question her own decision.

A player loves life and takes each challenge to find solutions that create the opportunities to work toward. To me it's like the parable of the talents in the book of Matthew in the Bible. Three men are given talents and asked to use them and multiply them. One man was given five and doubled them. Another was given two and doubled his. The man who was given one talent hid it in the ground. He was afraid to lose it and missed out on doubling it. Then he went full victim mentality. He complained about his lack of sleep and made excuses.

Nobody wants to marry a complainer who hides their best from the world. If you admire a person and want to get to know them better, find an opportunity to talk, plan an activity together, and learn from each other. You will either learn that you like certain personality traits or you will see there are certain personalities that you definitely don't want.

When you are looking for a spouse, you need to look at it as finding a teammate that will help you in life. Someone that will help you when you're down and you can help them when they are down. What is love? There are different types of love. At the beginning of young love, you may have a crush on someone and find them physically attractive. Over time, when you get to know the person and have experiences to draw you closer together, this becomes romantic love. But learning to be patient and kind through trials and challenges that test each of you and you stick together, this is real love. It will be hard, but remember, the grass is greener where you water it, so remember to do things for each other. Plan regular dates after you get married. Satan is going to try and break you up. He will try and put a wedge in between you and your spouse. It will start with little things and grow. Remember, it is Satan and his angels who do not want you to be happy.

You have control of you. Write down in your journal who you want to be. Work on being that person, and you'll attract the person you want by your example. When I was in high school, I had a crush who would not give me the time of day. We graduated and went our separate ways. I started focusing on the person I wanted to be and got involved in activities that interested me and helped me grow spiritually, physically, and emotionally. I was learning to love the person I was becoming. I found myself happy most of the time and loving life, and then my crush started to notice me. He came to a dance, and we reconnected, and soon we started dating. We had many good times together. We did not end up together because he went on a mission, and I let other girls misguide me with their gossip. The point is that when you develop yourself, feel confident in who you want to be, or just have a direction on where you want to go, that you will get noticed.

Also be kind. Boys can be shy too. It is nerve racking to ask a girl out. In fact, kindness above all other traits will give you and your spouse a long and happy marriage. If the other person has kindness, open up to them. If not, guard your heart.

You're worth it. Save yourself for someone who agrees.

CHAPTER II

Shape the Unknown Edges: How to Be a Homemaker Even if You're Not a Stay-at-Home Mom

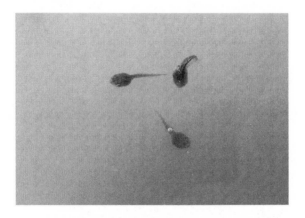

A word of encouragement during a failure is worth more than an hour of praise after success.

—Unknown

I always wanted to be a stay-at-home mom. Opportunities led me elsewhere. I did what I had to do to partner with my husband for my family, even if that meant going against the culture I grew up around: "to be a good mom you need to stay home with the kids."

Keith and I were a team. We were dealt a different lot in life than those who gave me that "advice" about motherhood. What we were able to do is make the kids' childhood *fun*. I had a fun childhood adventuring off into the red hills and I wanted to take the kids on adventures I had enjoyed. One of our favorite adventures was tadpole hunting in the spring down at the river. After work, we would grab a bucket and bacon or hot dogs and head to a park by the river. I would also pack a picnic dinner. The kids would run and play. Dig in the dirt. Use bacon and hot dogs to catch crawdads. As they would hunt they could find the shallow pools of water with the tadpoles which we called pollywogs. Sometimes we would take them home in a jar and see if we could keep them alive, but most of the time we would end up putting them back in the river. These small moments are actually the big moments in the kids' lives. It is not the amount of time we spend with the kids, it's the quality of time, love, and openness they feel.

The environment we create for our family is what is most important. On Saturday mornings my kids knew when it's time to clean. I cranked up the music and set a timer for thirty minutes. During the week if the house got too messy, I would set the timer for ten minutes. Let's see what we can get done. To their amazement, we usually got everything done. To them it was a game. It was for me too.

And that's what made life a challenge. How do I create quality time and be there for their big questions? I wanted to spend all my time with them . . . but couldn't. I wanted to explore and teach them, and help them find their answers to their curiosity. I could see their greatness and I wanted to help shape it. With evenings and weekends to learn and grow we learned how to work, explore, and figure things out. It helped them grow to take on responsibility and see the good Keith and I were doing to help others in our jobs. They learned quickly when Mom was serious. The moment I remember most is when we would go swimming, and we only had so much time. I would give a five-minute warning, and if they did not get out after the allotted time, I would not bring them back the next week. We had little snippets of adventures to make memories. It is important to take pictures. Life will pass by and it's easy to forget the fun. Print the pictures so the memories can keep the joy alive.

The little moments in life can leave a lasting impression and help to discover who you are.

I found out quickly that my oldest son loved biology and animals. He would lead the way to the best water hole or remind us to go on our adventures down to the river. He brought home any animal he could find and requested pets of the exotic. We were known as the neighborhood zoo. I was not fond of animals, but I knew how much he was learning and loved them.

My second son, Kyler, I learned, was more of a business kid. He really loved strategy, puzzles, and games. He would see the strategy quickly and beat us in our family game nights. He was the one to get us together and discover a new game.

My daughter wanted to do everything her brothers were doing. She always wanted to be involved with sports or activities that she was not old enough to join. She would beg and beg. She also loved working with her dad and wanted to be physically active. She was highly competitive, and sports were her love. When she was in sixth grade, she asked if there was a sports school, and if there was, she wanted to be shipped off to it. Obviously, I did not try too hard to find one. I would miss her too much and miss the opportunity to be her mom for the little time I had.

Let's talk about the little things you can do to make your time together better, especially if you don't get as much time with your kids as you'd like. Happy notes around the house can certainly cheer a person up and make a person feel loved. Eating dinner together is important as well. It gives everyone an opportunity to talk about their day and concerns they may have. We would talk about something that made them sad or worried and then talk about the best part of their day. We tried to leave on a good note and also give them the opportunity to talk about concerns.

Your example, what you are involved in, will help your children discover their gifts too. As an educator, I had a photography business on the side. This was part of our adventure too. We had to scout for good locations for the next photo shoot. I would also have my kids help me hold the reflector or camera equipment. Now my son is a better photographer than me. He picked up the details and lighting and brought in his own perspective.

When it came to birthdays, we really tried to make them memorable. Making an unusual cake sometimes worked out, and other times, it didn't. Food always brings people together and our family loves food. One of our favorite traditions that is small but memorable is making a cake or brownies every Sunday. The kids started making it when they got old enough to cook and read directions. Nothing beats a hot brownie with vanilla ice cream.

My father would visit his widowed mother every Monday. I know she loved it, and he did too. As I grew up, our tradition was to visit grandparents on Sunday. We need each other in our lives.

The top pick for my kids for memories was visiting their grandparents for the summers. They had the oldest bed-and-breakfast in Utah, which sat on nineteen acres. There was lots of work to do. They had guests who came to visit kids at the nearby college, golfers who planned a trip to the local eighteen-hole golf course, and campers who didn't want to camp when the rest of their family did. For two weeks, there was a big pageant that brought guests from all over the country to stay. My kids loved to go and help. They learned how to clean bathrooms, make beds, cook, and serve breakfast to guests. This was good not only for them but also for the grandparents. During the very little spare time that was available, the kids went adventuring or created items to sell to guests in the snack shop. As my husband's parents began to age, they needed more help, and eventually, they ended up selling the estate. Each one of my kids got the opportunity to learn from their grandparents and be a part of their lives. These are the times they will never forget.

At one point in my life, I worked in northern California and lived with my brother Roger; his wife, Hillary; and their kids. I realized the importance of dinner together and helping each other out with the simplest deed of having dinner ready. That one thought of not having to think about what to make for dinner relieved the stress for the day. Working all day and having dinner on the table helped set the tone of peace and relaxation in the house. It felt like I was running a race all day and the finish line was home with dinner. Thank you, Hillary!

Working moms have a hard time doing it all. Maybe set up a neighborhood dinner swap where you make a big batch of food to feed your family and another so they can have a day off. Then they do it in return. This can change up the dinner routine and give you a break too.

Most importantly, teach your kids to work. I strongly believe that every person should be industrious. Teach and give your kids opportunities to learn as young as you can. When my kids were eight, seven and three, Keith called to tell me he bought some land and we were going to build a house. I got panicky and nervous. How are we going to build a house? We have never done this on our own. My dad was a builder, and we had helped the family with remodeling, but to build one ourselves was nerve racking. *How will we pay for it? What is the process?* So many questions that we were going to have to figure out.

We spent nights working on a design. Keith figured out all the city planning items. We figured out what the bank needed so they could give us the construction loan, and we started digging in the dirt. We learned so much through the process. Keith got us organized and stayed on top of the paperwork from the subcontractors and their schedules. We would work our nine-to-five jobs in education and then grab pizzas and the kids and head over to the homesite. The subcontractors would do their work, and some would leave a mess. We gave the kids brooms, shovels, and whatever they needed to help us keep the site clean and to prepare for the next subcontractor to arrive in the morning. Some nights, we were there until midnight. The kids were a big help, and they realized all the hard work it takes to build a home. Once we moved in, we still had to put in the yard. The kids liked this part because they helped decide what we wanted to save for. We ended up putting in an outdoor drinking fountain and a basketball court area. I had my garden, and we picked different trees and flowers to put around the yard. These were fun days working together.

Maybe you do not have a good family relationship. Fill in with those you want to be with. Maybe there is an aunt or a neighbor, or you can adopt a grandmother who will let you into their lives. There is so much to learn from each other.

What are some of the traditions you would like to start? What are some of the routines you want to instill in your kids? My niece and her husband put their kids to bed at 7:00 p.m. and read the kids books for fifteen minutes before they fall asleep. This is great for my niece and her husband because they have time together after the kids are in bed. The kids are young and may or may not remember their conversations, but they will remember the bond they are building.

Decide now how you want to incorporate traditions into your life. Some will just fall in place. I love to travel. A few times, I got to take each child on their own little vacation with me for family events. My sister got married, and I took my youngest to her reception in Georgia. Another time, my brother was living in San Francisco, and I took the oldest there. I didn't want Kyler to miss out, so I scheduled a time for him to visit his uncle on another occasion. This soon led to planning adventures with each individually a couple of other times.

For many years, the kids wished I could be home with them, but now that they are older, they are glad for the time we did have together and the opportunity to see their mom work, which instilled a work ethic in them. They also see that it sometimes takes two incomes or more to survive. Remember, it is quality time not quantity time that matters. Even if you only do one adventure a month, write it down, put it on the calendar or on the fridge, and let the kids help plan it. It will all work out. Even if it doesn't at first. Or for a long while. In the end, *everything* works out.

CHAPTER 12

Fill the Barrel: How to Have Kids (And Not Mess Them Up)

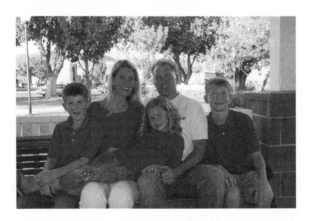

It's too easy to lose a diamond while you're busy collecting stones.
—Unknown

In high school, my friends and I attended Saturday night church dances. After the dances, most of us would go to the Macayo Mexican restaurant. Some would eat, and the rest of us would snack on the chips and salsa to enjoy good conversation, flirt, and catch up on the latest and greatest before heading home. My curfew was always midnight. A couple of times, I called and asked to stay out later, and my dad would always say, "Malissa, you have your free agency, and you know the consequences for not being in before curfew. You choose."

I always went home. I didn't want to suffer the consequences of losing my freedom to go to the dance the next week. I always appreciated my dad for letting me make my own decisions and also for reminding me of the consequences.

This chapter is not about parenting. Go read those books. This is about how to think about being a parent . . . and then do it without messing up your kids.

What type of parent do you want to be? Have you made a list or put a note in your journal? Many times I did. My mom would do something, and then I would say, "I'll never do that to my kids." Funny thing is that sometimes I have done what my mother did. Maybe for good reason and other times just from reaction.

Your parents aren't perfect, you won't be either, and neither was I. I must have missed Parenting 101! Even though I grew up in a family of nine, I am the second oldest and loved helping my mom most of the time. I thought I would be a great mom because I knew how to do everything. I would change diapers and clean the house, and I loved to cook. Just ask my siblings about the cooking. Still, to this day, they like it when I cook.

So when I was pregnant with my first child, I did not fret. I figured this would be a breeze, but when I brought Kaden home from the hospital, I was afraid. I remember the first diaper change. I panicked. This baby was mine. I was responsible. Did I remember how to change diapers? First of all, he was a boy, and he had this clip in his belly button area from the umbilical cord. I was worried I was going to hurt him. Luckily, my mom came into the room and helped me. It was a weird feeling knowing this child was mine. Once my mom started the diaper change, I felt relief, and it all came back to me.

Looking back, there are things I wish I had known or done differently. First, you can get pregnant while using birth control, and pregnancy affects everyone differently. Each time you are pregnant, you can have different symptoms. When I was pregnant with my boys, I threw up once in the middle of the night, and that was it. I was nauseated for the first trimester but didn't throw up unless it was on a crazy car ride. With my daughter, I threw up every day, and I gained the most weight with her. I could not figure out how I gained so much weight after all that came out.

When it was time to deliver my first child, he got stuck. My great baby-bearing hips were not the solution for easy deliveries as I had grown up thinking. The large, round Kelsch head and small birth canal made for complications. It was 2:00 a.m. when we arrived at the hospital, and they got me prepped. The doctor came in around 9:00 a.m. in his cowboy boots because he was called in from his ranch. This was a small town, and most people had farms and ranches.

Well, Kaden was stuck and needed assistance, so they tried the vacuum, but he did not budge. Then the doctor tried the forceps. On the first try, he slipped and fell back against the instrument tray, and the instruments flew all over the floor. This caused a loud ruckus, and I was scared. I thought the doctor had pulled off my baby's head. No one told me what to expect. I asked if the baby was all right, and the doctor said his head was out. Kaden had paved the way for his siblings. Now for the body. One more push and Kaden was born. They put him on my chest, and I looked at him. With all the pressure in the birth canal, the vacuum, and the forceps, he came out all bruised and with a sideways conehead. He was ugly. I thought to myself, *Do all babies come out this way?* I would soon find out. For months, his bruising and conehead remained. When we went out to meet up with friends, they would ask to see the baby and then turn to me and ask, "Are you OK?" I would not even get a fake "Oh, your baby is so cute."

If your baby looks weird, it's OK. My son is a brilliant gem now, so don't worry if yours come out as unpolished rocks.

Now that I had a baby, each time I wanted to go somewhere, it was a major event. I couldn't just grab my purse and head out the door. I had to go through the list. Bottles? Check Diapers? Check. Wipes? Check. Burp cloth? Check. Binky? Check. Blanket? Check. Car seat? Check. There was even more as they got to be a few months older. Then I needed toys and formula, and then sippy cups and snacks.

Once your child becomes a toddler, you have to grow eyes in the back of your head. They can be all over the place and into everything. If you have had a pet, you may know the feeling. If there is anything sacred, put it up high; otherwise, it will be eaten, ripped, or flushed down the toilet. Anything that can be put up a nose, in a mouth, or in an ear will be tried. Keep small objects away. Any electronics will be tested and hidden. The Magic Eraser was an amazing invention when my kids were small. It took the marker off my wood table and the walls. And when you turn around or take a shower, the kids will get into things you don't want them to. Nothing is safe.

I would classify early childhood as four-, five-, and six-year-olds. They are capable of many things. They can help around the house and even help with the dishes. Give them responsibilities. Let them help you, and let them watch. I remember my mother was the 4-H leader in our town, and she had the kids over. The one day that sticks in my memory is when she was teaching cooking. She had all the ingredients on the table and taught the 4-H kids how to read a recipe and what utensils to use when baking. I was an observer until she let me level off the flour as we made cookies. It was then that I learned I loved to cook and wanted to continue to learn. I was four, and I wanted to do more.

My kids learned to do the dishes, do yard work, and clean bathrooms. At this age they think it is fun to be an "adult" and want to play this game whenever you let them.

In middle childhood, they are still helpers, but they are learning that they want to do their own thing too. Then come the preteen years. Their bodies are changing and hormones raging. They become more of whatever personality they have. If they are shy, they get shier and are afraid to make a mistake or look like a fool in front of others. If they are an extrovert, they try to find more attention and want to hang out with friends or be in charge and lead the group. They all have insecurities as they try to find their way.

Teens think they know everything and are invincible. They think they can take on the world, and they don't need anyone, but they do. A friend of mine reminded me of the time she ran away from home to her friend's house. She went to school the next day and then went home.

She had forgotten she ran away and naturally went home the way she always did.

College or young adulthood can be fun and challenging at the same time. It is fun in the sense that you can have a conversation, and they are learning to think on their own. It's challenging that they are thinking on their own. They may not think what you think or do things the way you want or do yourself. You have to step back and let them make their own choices. They have free agency, and they have to learn from their mistakes and decisions.

What have you observed in your parents or their friends that you want to incorporate into your life as a parent? It's intentional parenting rather than doing what comes naturally, such as reacting in situations unproductively. Let the mothers you know or know of inspire you.

The mothers of several of my friends stood out to me when I was in high school. The first was Rebecca Cory. She was a popular and beautiful girl in our high school. What made her wonderful was that she was kind to everyone. She invited me and about ten others to her house for a get-together to watch a movie. I remember walking into the home; her mother greeted me so kindly and knew my name. She had a way of including a person and making them feel loved and welcomed. Another mom who made an impression was Terresa Hall's mom. One school day, she picked up Terresa to take her off campus for lunch. Terresa told her mom I was with her, and they invited me along. I had never had someone else's parent spend money on me for lunch. I realized then that I wanted to be like this mom and have special times with my daughter and her friends. Her generosity brought me close to her and was an example of what I wanted to do. I want my kids to see me as being generous and opening doors to anyone who needs it. I had many great examples in my life, and I'm so grateful for my friends who shared their families with me.

My favorite parenting example will always be my dad. Like he is, I want to be the sort of parent who is sorely missed when they are gone. Not just by the kids, but by cousins, siblings, community, and employees. I did not realize his reach until his passing. So many people came to visit after his death to tell me stories of how he had helped them in small and large ways. In my mind, I could see how he threw out pebbles of service into the big water of life, and the ripples were coming back to him, but he was not there to receive them. The family got to see them in his stead. And now, I think of what he told me after his passing: *Malissa, if I knew what I know now, I would not be afraid! Malissa, go for it. Be not afraid!* The fact that he did so many things and wanted to do more shows me there is a lot to do.

To be the best mother you can be, begin with the end in mind. Yes, you want to go into pregnancy, birth, and the early years equipped with useful information. Just as important is why. Set your purpose—you will be a mother whose love is cherished and missed for years after your passing. If you forget everything else, remember this. Decide today how you want to be remembered.

CHAPTER 13

Keep on Tumbling: How to Make Your Own Happy after Disappointment

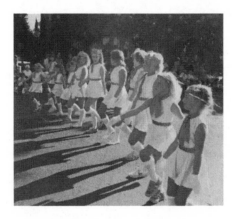

For every minute you are angry you lose sixty seconds of happiness.
—Ralph Waldo Emerson

In southern Utah back in the 1980s, the Super Stepper Drill Team was the group to be on. Tryouts for this dance and drill team were like tryouts for the football team for us girls. We'd show up at school with curlers in our hair so we would look perfect for the tryouts. All the girls, especially the popular girls, would be there. I wanted to be with the popular girls.

The week of tryouts, we had practice every day to learn the routine. It was hard work. By the time practice was done, I was hot, sweaty, and thirsty. My mom would pick me up and ask how it went. I thought I was doing really well. I felt I would make the team and be with the popular girls. I could not wait.

Tryouts came, and they went well. I did the best I could. We would find out that night with a phone call whether I made the team or not. When the call came, it was a call of unfortunate results. I did not make it. Oh, the shame I would feel the next day at school. I was not cool. I ran to my room and cried. Later, after I had calmed down, my mom came to my room and asked if I wanted to be on another drill team. I had no idea what she was talking about. She said she would create one, and I could ask all my friends who didn't make the Super Steppers if they wanted to be on our team. I was so excited. I said yes. The next day at school was a day of excitement. Who would be on the team with me? I went through the halls and asked everyone how they did in the tryouts. If they had not made the team, I asked them to be on mine. We had girls of all shapes and sizes, and it was fun. We practiced every day. When it was time for the parades, we got to wear our hair in curlers to school. I remember that first parade. It was so hot. The parade route was about a mile long, and we had to march the whole way. At the end, we were exhausted, but we shone. We were all thrilled to be able to perform. We had many other parades but only lasted one year as the Starlettes. Most of us made the second most desirable team, the Dixie Dazzlers, the next year.

My mom really showed me how to turn my disappointments around and see the possibilities. She believed in making your own opportunities, and I am thankful for her teaching me this. It has helped me many times in my life.

Have you had a disappointment that turned into something even better? Many times, we think we have to have something a certain way and are unaware there is a better path for us.

I always wanted a big family. One of my major disappointments and a change of plans occurred when my family was young, and I thought I was pregnant. I tested myself several times that week, and each morning, the test came up negative. I started to get a little belly. First thing in the morning, I would see this little belly, then I would go to the restroom, and it would shrink. I watched my belly for several weeks, but on the first Saturday in October 2002, it did not shrink. This little round belly stayed, so I took another pregnancy test, and it came up negative. I got scared this time and went to the ER. The trip was a little hectic because we had the Saint George Marathon on this weekend every year, and they had the roads blocked and runners on their way to the finish line.

When I got to the hospital, the doctors thought I was pregnant. They did their tests, and sure enough, I was not pregnant. They were concerned and did more testing and X-rays. There it was: a tumor the size of a cantaloupe growing fast. It had latched on to a blood supply, and they were afraid it would grow too fast and burst, and I would hemorrhage and die before I could get medical help. They recommended and scheduled surgery right away. I told them if they could save my uterus, please do. I wanted to have more children. The doctor said he would if he could.

I came out of surgery, and the first question I asked the doctor was "Can I have more kids?" He told me no. He was not able to save my uterus. I recovered, but my heart ached. I did not get to choose this result. I had wanted a big family like the one I grew up in. I counted the three blessings I had already—my kids. At least I got three, and I decided to run the Saint George Marathon to replace the loss and remember that I am alive and healthy.

I may not have personally received more children, but I have had the opportunity to be a part of the lives of many children through the primary program and especially Young Women organizations in our church.

Even when life doesn't offer you what you asked for, you can still make the best of it. That's why we all know the old saying about lemons and lemonade. We innately know we have to make the best of it. And we get to choose.

Maybe you are thinking of a plan that did not go your way. The puzzle is to see what opportunities are nearby. Are you missing opportunities because you are caught up in your original plan for how it was supposed to be or what you wanted? Let's look at what you can do to take courage and go for another opportunity. I'm giving you permission to dream big. Look for the barrel that will shape you into the person you want to be. Step into that barrel to get yourself tumbling, even if it is on the sidelines. At least you're in the barrel, and you're working toward making your own happy.

Think of some disappointments. Things you really wanted or experiences you wished you'd had, but it's too late now. How did everything turn out? What turned out better than you thought it would? Is there anything you can do to make the best of it, like volunteering with children when you wish you'd had more?

Sometimes, making your own happiness is a matter of taking one step at a time. The tumbling may take longer than you think, but keep tumbling your rocks. Because that is how rocks are polished smooth.

In the late nineties, when I was the young mother of two boys, I started looking for work to cover our medical expenses. I looked in the newspaper and saw a fundraising job at the University of Utah. I was so excited to apply because I had started many fundraising events and raised a good amount of money for a small-town girl. I felt very qualified for the position.

Weeks went by without any word. At the time, I did not realize how long it takes to get a job in education. One day, I got up the courage to go to the university and introduce myself to the director. I got lucky that day, and he was in. He was kind enough to invite me into his office and ask me questions about myself and my experience. I told him I had applied for the major gifts position. He came right out and told me I did not have enough experience. I was shocked. I'd been sure I was qualified. What a disappointment.

To my astonishment, he actually offered me a job as his assistant. His former assistant had just left for another job, and HR had not sent him anyone yet. I was thrilled. If I could not have the job I wanted because of my lack of experience, then the next best thing would be to be in the department that I could learn and grow in. This would lead to the experience I would need and introduce me to a whole new world I never could have imagined. During my time as the assistant to the major gifts director, I planned events all over the country for the president of the university, the director of major gifts, and all the major gift officers.

I helped raise money for scholarships and buildings. I was part of the team that remodeled and built Gardner Hall on Presidents Circle at the University of Utah. In honor of all my hard work, there is a book in the music library in Gardner Hall that is dedicated to me with my name in it. The experience was amazing. It taught me the power of investing in my professional development by allowing me to go to seminars that I was interested in. This all came to pass because I had the courage to drive to the university, to ask, and to see the opportunity that was different from what I wanted. Have the courage to dream big, and if you don't make it your first time, see what door opens along the way. Trust that at least one will open—and it will.

CHAPTER 14

Show Off Your Shine: How to Love Yourself into Self-Confidence

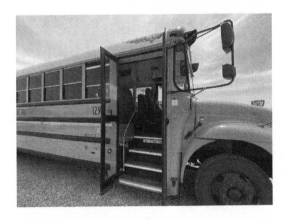

I destroy my enemies when I make them my friends.
—Abraham Lincoln

It was a dark, cold, wintery night around 6:00 p.m. I was traveling down a two-way highway in my minivan. It was dark, and the lights of the vehicles coming at me in the northbound lane were bright. I had the radio on, playing an eighties station. I was dancing in my seat to the music. The traffic was heavy, and I was enjoying my ride home from a long day at work at the University of Utah. I was pregnant and could not wait to get home and relax. All of a sudden, I felt my grandmother's presence. She had died six years earlier in a car accident. In my mind, she told me, *Turn the radio off! Malissa, pay attention to the road.* I was shocked to feel and hear her, so I did exactly what she said. Moments later, a large truck approached from the right side into my lane without stopping. I had to swerve into northbound traffic to miss the truck and then had to speed up and get back in my lane so as not to be hit by northbound traffic. If I had not listened to my grandmother's spirit, the situation would have been fatal.

We have angels all around us if we just listen. Here's ways I've found that you can improve your ability to hear them. First, turn off distractions—radio, TV, music, social media. Second, notice suggestions that quietly come across your mind. If they uplift you or bring hope to you or others, accept them. Third, if they contain a warning, heed it.

Even when you feel all alone, there are forces at work on your behalf. The Lord loves you and wants you to succeed. He wants you to feel loved. You are a daughter of God. You have a Divine Nature that God wants you to realize, uncover, and let shine. He doesn't want you to do it alone. We are all here to bump up against each other through the grit of life and brush off the jagged edges. The process of struggle and discovery is the path to reveal your Divine Nature and the character within you. You need to find people here in person to love and be loved.

Three living angels reached out to me at a low point in my life. Keith and I had sold the house we built and found a little fixer-upper home out of town. I remember thinking, *There are many second homes and cabins here; no one will find me.* I wanted to hide from the world. Then there were three women: Kathy, Karen, and Kaylynn. They were in charge of the Young Women in this area and called me to help them. I agreed, but I thought they didn't really need me, so I didn't care if they included me. They did call, and they did always include me. They reached out in more ways than a church calling. They really wanted to be my friend. At this time in my life, when I wanted to hide away, they reached out to keep me tumbling. They are amazing great friends to this day. They have genuine hearts and are living examples of love and kindness. We became a true sisterhood. They supported me spiritually when I was ready to give up and reminded me that God loves us all in every season of our lives.

Embracing Self-Confidence

You will find this chapter a little different from the previous ones you've read. Raising, teaching, mentoring, and knowing girls from all backgrounds, I've realized that Christ-centered self-confidence is the most important trait a young woman can possess. Believe in God and believe in yourself, and you will naturally take good care of yourself, accept the responsibility of adulthood, develop useful skills, surround yourself with lovely people, and mature spiritually. That's why I will be offering step-by-step guidance in subsequent sections of this chapter. These activities and advice will help you release anti-confidence (I'll tell you shortly what that is) so you can experience everything God desires for you.

Now, with this trait—self-confidence—being so important, we ought to define it before we go any further. Self-confidence comes when you realize you are loved by God always, just as you are. You can reveal your character by doing good in the world and learning new things. Spend the time you need in the morning to fix yourself so you feel pretty. As soon as you walk out the door, turn your focus outward by sharing and using your talents. Include others who may feel alone. A quick way to earn friends is to compliment everyone on the things you see that are good.

Remember, you are an individual, and the Lord wants you to develop your talents. He sees your infinite potential. He loves you, and he wants you to find joy. So what brings you joy? Let's find out.

List five things that bring you joy.

1. _____
2. _____
3. _____
4. _____
5. _____

While writing this book, I dreamed I missed the bus like the ten virgins who didn't have their oil lamps full when the groom arrived. I was heartbroken and overwhelmed with anxiety and depression. I had been doing so many good things, and now I had missed the bus. Satan wanted me to give up. Satan wants you to feel discouraged in what you are doing. He doesn't want you reading and gaining strength and encouragement to better yourself and be a tool for the Lord. He will try every mind game to take you out. That's why we all need backup. If you don't have someone physically near you, reach for an uplifting book, a podcast, music, church, a social group. The day I wrote this chapter, I got my pep talk from a podcast. So who is your backup team?

List five people or resources that can pick you up when you feel down.

1. _____
2. _____
3. _____
4. _____
5. _____

Seek to serve others and spread some sunshine. When I was in high school and felt discouraged and depressed, I would go to the flower shop, buy two dozen roses, and pass them out to random people. I figured if I was having a hard time, who else was too? I thought about what would brighten my day, and flowers always came to mind. As I gave away a single-stem rose, people would light up and be surprised. This brought joy to them and helped me break out of the storm that was in my mind. It didn't always work perfectly to get me out of the depression, but taking action gave me experience, strengthened my faith, and opened a vehicle for God to teach me.

The Confidence-Jealousy Connection

A lack of self-confidence often manifests not only as self-doubt but also as jealousy, what I call anti-confidence. Feeling envious of another is a sign that we feel we're missing something, that we're missing out, that we're messing up compared to other people.

One beautiful spring afternoon when I was twelve, I hopped on the school bus for home. I sat near the middle, as usual, and the popular girls, Sarah, Brooke, and Debbie, sat behind me. They told me how much they adored my clothes—how cute I looked today. I felt relieved because my jeans and blouse had come from a thrift store. My family did not have a lot of money, but that day, I measured up. I thought the popular girls wanted to be my friends!

My bus stop was second to the last on the route, and my new pals got off at the stop before mine. When it was my turn, I got up and headed toward the door. The kids who were still on the bus giggled as I passed. I didn't stop to ask why. I just hurried off and ran toward my younger cousin, who had just gotten off the bus before me.

"Malissa!" she called out to me. "Come here!"

"What?"

"What's that taped to your back?"

"What?"

Then I reached back and found them—notes that said "Kick me" taped on my back.

Those girls . . . they didn't want to be my friends. They didn't even like me. They just wanted to make fun of me. Had they been planning their prank all day? Why me?

I dragged myself home. Those mean girls popped my confidence like a balloon.

Months later, after keeping my distance, a classmate told me they were just jealous because a boy Debbie was chasing liked me instead.

A couple of years later, my family moved from small-town Utah to big-city Las Vegas. It was the middle of the school year. Junior high is awkward enough. Now I was a stranger with no friends, and everyone else was already settled into their cliques.

Woodbury Junior High was big, with over 1,500 students and what felt like that many different backgrounds, cultures, religions, and races. My hometown was the Shire—a little village where everyone looks and lives basically the same and knows everyone else's business. We had what seemed like five hundred students in the whole school district.

I was looking forward to meeting new people and learning how other kids grew up, what their family's traditions were, and what foods they ate. But I was shy, so I waited for someone else to make the first move. That was Stacey in first-period typing class. She asked the usual questions.

"So what's your name? Where are you from? What do you like to do?"

I answered and repeated her questions back to her.

Then she offered to look at my schedule and gave me the lowdown on the teachers. I thanked her.

At lunch, Stacey invited me to her table. The other girls at the table filled me in on the boys in our grade and who already liked who. There were still a few cute boys no one had spoken for yet, so I looked forward to getting to know them.

This excitement kept up for my first couple of weeks. I loved the attention. But there was this one girl who did not like me. Kami. I saw her in the school gym one day. She looked nice: tall, thin, short blonde hair. Word got around that she hated me, and we hadn't even met.

Stacey finally found out and told me why—because a boy Kami liked, liked me instead.

For months, gossip about "that new girl from Utah" spread around school. I eventually traced the rumors back to Kami. She wanted me to be an outcast. The school's various cliques divided—you had to like Kami or me.

The turning point was a multi–church group girl's camp. Our families were members of the same church but attended at different locations. The Young Women's leaders assigned Kami and me to collaborate on a project. At first, that felt impossible. Our very brief conversations were "strictly business." But the deeper we got into the work, the more we *had* to talk. Soon we found out what else we had in common besides school and church.

It turned out that our sisters were already friends. And we both liked to be creative. I liked art; Kami liked to write. She liked to dance. So did I. She told me about some cool new music she was listening to—U2, Depeche Mode, the Thompson Twins. Then one day, Kami loaned me a few of her favorite cassettes. That same day, she apologized for how she had treated me: for gossiping about me and uniting half the school against me, all over a boy who, as junior high crushes go, Kami had gotten over.

We became best friends.

Eventually, Kami and I made a pact never to let a boy get in the way of our friendship.

Prior to their seasons of jealousy, Debbie and Kami were both probably lovely girls. That changed when envy took over, when they wanted what they thought someone else had. At that age, clothes and boys are the usual triggers, but jealousy can creep in at any age, especially when we feel sorry for ourselves.

When Keith and I got married, we lived with his grandmother in a mobile home as we fixed up the basement the trailer was sitting on. You know the scene from *Indiana Jones and the Temple of Doom* where Harrison Ford walks through the curtains of webs and rats and darkness? That was what I was moving into in the basement. Just add plumbing pipes exposed in the ceiling, and you've got the picture. There was no kitchen or cabinets, just a dirty bathroom. We're roll-up-your-sleeves-and-get-to-work kind of people, and we saw potential. Our first task for the remodel was to clean up. When we took a load of trash to the dump, we found a kitchen sink, brought it home to our gloomy basement, and installed it ourselves. My best friend from college came to visit and saw that I had no cabinets, and her father was getting rid of the ones in his garage, so they gave them to us. Slowly, we put our little basement home together and made it cozy.

My daughter Makinzie's story was entirely different. And I have to admit . . . I felt jealous. Her soon-to-be husband wanted to buy her a *brand new* home. I was going down the rabbit hole of envy, but for two days, I was distraught because I could not admit this. I just wanted to be frustrated. As humans, it takes time for us to be tested, refined, and polished—ugh. The hardest part is admitting it. I did not want to say it. But as soon as I said it out loud and realized what I was thinking, I felt the release and could start to get back on track.

These stories were one-on-one, in-person experiences. Now, with the internet, we can be jealous of people around the world. We see glimpses into other people's lives at amazing times, all at once, which can quickly make us feel inadequate. Jealousy can lead to bullying as we can see from the stories. Now bullying has gone online. We can be bullied by people we don't even know from towns, cities, and countries we have never been to.

Bless those who hate you, to paraphrase scripture. One way to combat the situation, depending on the level of hate they have, is to delete the comment, be kind, and flip the situation to talk about them in a positive light and to help them notice their gifts and talents. Also, realize that they are the ones feeling inadequate.

Some people are looking for reasons to be outraged, and you can't change them. You can only change yourself and your environment. If things are getting out of hand, remove yourself from the situation. Realize that if you post something on social media, it can be found and will last forever on the internet. It will stay with you. It can be looked up. Bullying is not OK. If you cannot say something nice, do not say anything at all. With social media, we see everyone's one moment of happiness, not their whole life and how they are getting tumbled. We see the one side of a person that seems to be smoothed out and glorious, but they have rough edges that they are working on too.

If you are bullying others, *stop it* right now. If you are being bullied, please let someone know. You are a daughter of God and have a Divine Nature. You are amazing.

Let's celebrate each other's wins. God is asking us to love one another. Have empathy. Give grace. Share genuine compliments. These are some of the ways to fight jealousy and build your confidence. Let's dive a little deeper.

Tips to Replace Jealousy with Self-Confidence

Confidence is not created in a vacuum—we can't just retreat to our bedroom, get ready to face the world, and step out feeling confident.

Jealousy doesn't work that way either. Neither is something you do; they're the *result* of what you do, specifically, in the presence of others.

So I'm not going to tell you, "Just be more confident and less jealous." That would be obvious and also useless. Instead, you'll learn some effective strategies that, when followed, *result* in a greater sense of confidence in yourself and a lessened or even totally depleted feeling of jealousy.

To that end, with these tips, you can begin with yourself and finish with others who are in your life or who you want to be in your life through books, podcasts, or in actual real life. What all these tips have in common is how you treat others—and how you allow them to treat you.

■ Release Criticism

Self-criticism is the most destructive. It usually shows up when you are comparing yourself to someone else or maybe yourself. Your self-talk brings you down the quickest. When I received my patriarchal blessing at age fourteen (an ordinance within the Church of Jesus Christ of Latter-day Saints), I was told, "Think good thoughts, and you'll do good deeds."

My life experience since then has proved that true. Your subconscious listens to every word you say, so fill it with good thoughts. Have you ever watched how lovingly people talk to a baby? A sweet voice and encouragement. If the little one attempts to talk or walk, people are happy the baby even tried. What if we gave that same self-talk to ourselves?

Replace the self-talk about all your mistakes with words of encouragement. Here are some examples:

I am loved by a Heavenly Father and Mother.

I have divine qualities.

There is only one me.

I'm good enough.

I'm courageous.

I'm smart.

I'm responsible.

I love to smile.

Today's my lucky day!

I got this!

Write down the short pep talk you'll give yourself when negative thoughts creep in. I suggest turning the unhelpful self-talk inside out into its opposite—a helpful, positive affirmation: _____

_____

▪ Recognize Fears

What is driving you to think these thoughts? Are you feeling not good enough or that something is not fair? Maybe you're afraid of not being liked? Are you trying to keep up instead of looking at the path that is yours? Fear is usually the first cause. If you narrow down the fear, then you can change your thoughts and move forward with faith. It is one step at a time.

▪ Acknowledge

Jealousy is normal. It's what you do after you realize you are jealous that counts. Recognizing and acknowledging feelings of jealousy are the doors to self-confidence. As soon as you realize what feelings are affecting you, they can subside and reduce the emotion. I could have turned around and started saying bad things about the girls who were mean and not treating me fairly, but what would that have solved? Nothing. Take the higher example and show love. Understand that they are hurting just like you are hurting when you are jealous.

▪ Count Your Blessings

Always . . . no matter what . . . no matter how hard it gets . . . if you dig deep, you *will* find the good in you. Just take a baby step. If you have to ask someone close to you what you are good at, please do. Grab hold of the one or many things you have to be grateful for. Write a note to someone. There are people in my life I admire because they can turn negative things into something funny, and it lightens the mood. My husband's architect inspires me. He used to be a framer, but he had a biking accident, broke his spine, and is a paraplegic. He thinks about actor Christopher Reeve, the first Superman, who broke his neck, lost the use of his entire body, from his nose down, and could not even talk. Every day, Keith's colleague is grateful for the use of his shoulders and his arms so he can be an architect and provide for his family.

■ Pray for Strength

You can pray anywhere. Go out in nature. Go for a walk. Watch the birds. Be alone and pray for an eternal perspective. Ask and you shall receive. The Lord wants to help you. He loves you. When you pray, remember to thank the Lord first, ask for forgiveness, ask for what you need, and agree to follow His ways. I hope this gives you a guideline for prayer.

■ Build Boundaries

Understanding boundaries and enforcing them are vital skills that are not talked about much. When I was growing up, no one told me how to set boundaries and hold to them. Sometimes, my friends talked me into doing things I did not want to do, and then I regretted them and held animosity toward my friends. If you only say yes out of guilt or because you are worried about what people think, then the answer should be no.

Here is a simple, nonconfrontational way to build boundaries so you're able to keep your free agency without offending your friend: "That's not going to work for me. Thanks for asking." Or "Let me get back to you." Practice these phrases so you are ready when the answer is no or you need more time to think. Also, you do not have to give any explanation; just stick to repeating the phrase if they persist.

Having boundaries for jealousy means deleting hateful comments on social media sites, stepping out of a room to calm down if someone is speaking unkindly, and remembering that the person who is jealous is hurting. Have empathy and be kind.

▪ Befriend Trustworthy People

Surround yourself with genuine people. You know: the person who loves you even when you make a mistake, the person you can talk to and express your feelings. They always have an open mind to you. They want to help when they can.

As you build a small group of girlfriends who know, like, and trust each other, you'll find yourselves forming a sisterhood. That word has gone out of style, but I'm bringing it back. Recently, I gave a presentation about sisterhood for the Relief Society. I told all the young ladies that sisterhood means more than friendship. It's a bond between women who share common goals, lift each other up, and strive together to become more Christlike in every area of life. They encourage one another because of shared values and the unshakeable trust they have in one another. Jealousy has no place in a sisterhood because a win for one girl is a win for everyone.

▪ Give Love Freely

Love is interesting. We think of it as a feeling, but it's really an action. When you give it, it comes back multiplied, and it doesn't cost you anything. If it is not received, you can still feel good because you did the right thing. To be happy for another person will free your spirit. I have found that it's easier said than done, but just the thought can give you the courage to act and give love. Telling someone "I love you because . . ." fills their bucket and yours too. I have discovered when I notice the good in others and express my love for them, not expecting anything in return, I receive a sense of freedom.

▪ Always Ask for Forgiveness

You will be stronger when you can forgive. It takes the heavy burden of carrying the rock and lets it go. It frees your spirit. Asking for forgiveness for jealousy gives you the power to march ahead to build one more layer of strength and self-confidence. You are wise because you recognized, and you are strong because you followed through and corrected wrongs. Knowing you made it through the process builds confidence. The more you work on it, the stronger you will become.

■ Be Generous

The first living example of generosity I recall outside my family is a friend's mom. She made us cookies as we girls played tea party. Then there was a neighbor who gave my sister and me knee-high white patent-leather boots so we could be trendy in the seventies. Later came Terresa's mom, who took me to lunch. Then Sweetie with all her projects that gave our family extra income. Phil and Tami on a night out for our family. A neighborhood coming together to be a secret Santa. Several bosses gave generously to our team for industry-best systems and software so we can all be successful at work. Coworkers and friends who give whenever asked to support a good cause. And the many smiles that brightened my day. The list could fill this book.

I've noticed that those who give have a strong sense of self-confidence because they feel abundant. From the small actions of generosity to the large ones, you never know when you will make a difference.

The best example of generosity we have is Christ himself. He gives more than enough. When he turned water into wine for the wedding party, it was the best and more than enough. When Simon needed to pay his taxes, the Lord blessed him with a large net of fish that filled his boat and another.

List five ways you can show generosity today.

1. _____
2. _____
3. _____
4. _____
5. _____

■ Make Memories

When a mistake happens and is forgiven, the relationship is absolutely worth saving. Restart fresh right away. Create new happy memories together as soon as possible, even if it's awkward. Push through the awkwardness and rebuild your relationship. Kami and I became best friends because we chose to make happy memories together.

■ Remember You Are Never Alone

The avoided car crash wasn't the first time I've heard a voice. One of my earliest memories is from when I was eight years old and lived in Las Vegas. I had a friend who lived several blocks away. One day, we were in her front yard playing Barbies in a large mulberry tree that had been shaped to have the big, strong branches grow out with a slight platform in the center where we could both sit. I got an uneasy feeling and knew it was getting close to time to go home. My mom was very strict about me being home exactly at 5:00 p.m. I felt that I should not go home yet, but I was afraid of my mother getting mad and maybe worrying where I might be. As we began to clean up, I noticed two young men in a car parked in front of the house next door. I watched them for maybe ten minutes. They were both in the car, and then one would go into the house. He would come out, and the other went into the house. At one point, they were both in the house, so we hopped down from the tree to take the Barbie toys into the house to put them away. As I was leaving my friend's house, I hoped the young men had left because I had to walk in that direction to get home. As I left, I could see they were still in the house next door, so I walked briskly by, keeping my head down. As soon as I walked past their house and around the corner, a voice told me to hide. I thought, *Nothing is going to happen. That only happens in the movies or on TV. I am just paranoid.* Again, the voice said, *Hide, Malissa!* Again, I thought my mind was playing tricks on me. As I passed the corner backyard fence to the next backyard fence, I saw a tamarisk bush. I heard the voice again: *Malissa, hide in the bush!* I thought that even if I hid in the bush, they'd see my feet. *Nothing will happen to me.* I passed the bush. Just as I passed that tamarisk bush, those young men came screeching around the corner in their car yelling, "Get the girl! Get the girl!" One of the boys was going to jump out of the car to grab me.

I was afraid and started running. I could not believe they were really after me. I ran as hard as I could. Luckily, I loved to run, and I ran and ran. I ran around the corner and through a yard and made a U-turn to get back to my friend's house as they tried to turn around in their car. I made it back to my friend's house, and I pounded on the door. Her mom opened the door, saw my panic, and quickly pulled me in. She hugged me and asked what was going on. I told her what had happened, and she called the police. I was shaking when they interviewed me. I stayed for a while longer, and my friend's mom called my mom to let her know why. When I had calmed down, my friend and her big sister walked me home the long way in the other direction. The boys were picked up by police later that night and arrested for drug use.

Remember, you have people and angels who want to protect you. Listen to the small voice that can protect and guide you, both when you are in physical danger and those times you're feeling the inner turmoil of jealousy.

Baby steps. The very next time you feel down on yourself, like that other girl is *so much* better than you, return to this book. Flip open the tips. Pick the one you find easiest, and try it immediately. Then the next time, the best way to respond to self-doubt and its companion, jealousy, will come to you naturally.

Soon, you won't even need to pick this book up and reread this chapter.

Because it worked.

CHAPTER 15

Prepare for Final Polish: How to Have an Eternal Perspective

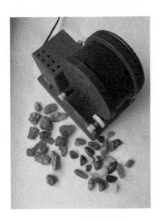

The happiness of your life depends upon the quality of your thoughts.
—Marcus Aurelius

I remember the day my daughter and I got our first pedicure together. It was a beautiful spring afternoon, and we thought it was time to let our toes break out of their dusty work shoes and make their appearance for the season. For Christmas, I bought the kids' experiences instead of actual physical gifts. There were so many things in this world to try that I thought we better get going and start experiencing the world, and a pedicure was on the list. I also figured it would be a good idea to spend time together and talk about what's on her mind. We got to the day spa early and talked about her day and the excitement of a job offer. She told me of some of her goals and what she was excited about and her future plans. Then she asked me a question: "How do you keep an eternal perspective? How do you know if you are caught up in the world?" I didn't get to answer her right away because the nail tech came to take us to our seats.

What a deep thought and a challenge to answer, and here is my reply:

You do *not* have an eternal perspective when your love for worldly items and processes are greater than your love for your Heavenly Father's ways. When you are given a choice and you pick the worldly one that only benefits you and don't look at the eternal consequences. Keep God in your mind. Is this what He would want you to do? Have an eye toward heaven and love your Heavenly Father and Jesus Christ. Recognize His strength and His ways. If you care more about what people think than what God thinks, then this will be a sign of going against an eternal perspective. If the love of money and worldly possession takes a stronger hold than helping a neighbor, this is another sign of being caught up in the world. Love one another. Love your neighbor. And always remember to pray.

What does this eternal perspective look like in practice? Daily prayer, for one. If you don't know how to pray, that's OK. Simply start by sharing what you are grateful for, repenting of weaknesses, asking for His strength, and agreeing to do His will when there is a choice placed before you.

Another way to adopt the eternal perspective is treating people right. Here in the real world, prioritizing your relationship with God manifests in the way you treat his greatest creation—other human beings. Both in the church and out, we generally recognize that true, lasting beauty is found not in the way a woman looks, but in how she conducts herself. Women known for faith, hope, and charity attract exactly that in return. Good people want to be around other good people. Christlike kindness and character cannot be faked.

To live the best earthly life possible—to make the most of every moment you're given—keep these three sisters close: faith, hope, and charity.

Why these three? Larry Hiller's talk "Hope: The Misunderstood Sister" discusses these three within the sister analogy. It meant a lot to me, and I'm sure it will bless you too.

First there is Faith. Everyone wants to hang around her. She is out-going and ready to make things happen. Even if you don't think it can be done, she is the one that gets it done. She is creative and likes to try new things.

> Now faith is the substance of things hoped for, the evidence of things not seen.
> —Hebrews 11:1

> Faith is not to have a perfect knowledge of things; therefore if ye have faith ye hope for things which are not seen, which are true.
> —Alma 32:21, Book of Mormon

True faith always moves its possessor to some kind of physical and mental action. If we take the rock tumbler as our metaphor, then getting in the bucket is faith. And from faith we then see miracles. As a note on the process of the tumbling, repentance is the water washing away the jagged edges that have broken off.

Second is Hope. She is confident and quiet with a peaceful walk. She has experienced hardship, loss, and great trials, but she still looks to the future with brightness. She takes her time and is steady. When there are days of darkness and the path seems lost, Hope keeps moving forward and holds our hand. She keeps us going.

Hope is the churning of the bucket to keep moving forward. Hope is feeling the pain of the jagged edges being removed and keeping going, knowing you're moving forward toward Christ.

Hope is not hardening your heart. If you stop the rock tumbler and don't clean it out and continue the process, everything will harden inside the barrel. You need to keep churning.

Third is Charity. She is humble, beautiful, and kind. You can feel her love when you are in her presence. You feel accepted for who you are at this very moment. She waits patiently for you to come along with her and be her buddy. She knows what you need before you ask and steps in to lift you up. She handles things with grace and generosity. All want to be in her presence.

There are two ways to look at charity: vertically and horizontally. Vertically, it is the love Christ has for us. It is our connection to heaven and the atonement. Horizontal charity is the love we have for our neighbor and how we treat one another here on earth.

Brett G. Scharffs further explains charity in three ways. First, by the way we listen and seek to understand one another. We are all doing the best we can.

Second, by the way we give, serve others, and lift or boost another. It may be easy to bring someone up, but can we lift another person above us? When I feel jealous, it is because I think it is unfair that another person is being boosted above me. For example, I worked hard to build my business, and I trained someone else, and she got the promotion. This was hard. I look at the pioneers and how they sacrificed, and their sacrifice has boosted me above their circumstances.

Third is the way we love and care for others.

> Wherefore, my beloved brethren, if ye have not charity, ye are nothing, for charity never faileth. Wherefore, cleave unto charity, which is the greatest of all, for all things must fail—
>
> But charity is the pure love of Christ, and it endureth forever; and whoso is found possessed of it at the last day, it shall be well with him.
>
> —Moroni 7:46–47, Book of Mormon

Charity is how we bump up against each other.

Grit of Life

We can choose to put people in our lives to grind our rough edges. Life also throws some grit in the barrel to shape us. The more difficult a situation—the grittier the grit—the more important it is to let faith, hope, and charity guide you. In their absence, you may find yourself lost on a dark path. I speak from experience.

The following story will be surprising to a lot of people who know Keith and me. To our community, friends, and family, we seem to have a good marriage and great kids. And the reason we do is because we outlasted seasons of life like this one.

It was my husband's birthday, and I had decorated the house. Family would be there soon to join in the celebration. The food was made, the presents wrapped, and the candles on the cake. I remember going through the motions, but I had had it. I was done with this relationship. I was tired of being broke, working outside the home, and taking care of the kids. I figured I could do it on my own and didn't need him. Heck, I was doing it already. We were by the front door ready to let people in, and that's when I told him I wanted a divorce. The party started, and we pretended to be happy. I don't know what Keith was thinking or if he even heard me, but in my mind, I was going through what I had to do to separate myself and get on my own. Bank accounts to separate. Bills to separate, living conditions to separate. We didn't talk about it. That night when I knelt to pray, the words came to my mind: *Malissa, you have your free agency to choose. Choose wisely.*

The next day, I went to the bank and started the process. I had just left the bank, and a friend called me up. She asked me how I was doing. I gave the typical "Fine," and we talked some more. Finally, I told her what I was doing at the moment, and she told me not to go through with it. She said she rarely got strong impressions, but she had a strong feeling to call me and tell me to stop whatever I was going to do. We talked about all that I had been through, and she lovingly listened and then repeated that I shouldn't go through with it. I listened carefully to her words and took another moment to think through what I was about

133

to do. My next stop was an attorney. I decided to go to work and think it through some more. The words came to my mind again: *Malissa, you have your free agency to choose. Choose wisely.*

I began to think about how mountains were moved to get Keith and me together. There was a plan bigger than me and my selfish desires. I began to look at the eternal consequences of this decision. *Keith has a good heart. He doesn't have an addiction. He has always been faithful to me. He is not abusive. He keeps his covenants of marriage. Why can't I make this work?* I was maxed out.

What was actually bothering me? My pride and frustration—they were blinding me. Satan wanted me to blame my husband for everything. It's Satan's plan to break up the family, any family, *every* family. He had gotten a wedge into our marriage through me and was about to cause a split. I reflected on the pioneers and all they had gone through. Their love and bonds kept them together, and they had it harder than I did. If they could get through their suffering, surely I could.

I decided to cancel my plans to divorce, work through my issues, and work on us. The adage "The grass is greener where you water it" came to my mind, and I decided to create a different plan. An eternal plan.

This was a hard story to tell. I do want to help women get through the struggle when they think it's too hard, and they can't take it anymore or think they can do it on their own. I think women need support in this area. We have to work and balance everything. It is hard on men trying to navigate the world too. Not everyone is lucky in jobs and opportunities. How can we have more love and kindness toward our spouses?

There are going to be rough times, and with a teammate to go through life with, you'll have more strength than you'd have alone. Things are not always going to go the way you plan. I have found people are not always going to agree with what you think, but be kind and remember that we are all spiritual beings with bodies to have experiences on earth that shape us and help us grow into the faith, hope, and charity Heavenly Father desires for us. Through faith, we know things will get better—even if we don't see how. With hope, we do the right thing because it's the right thing. And because of charity, we expect nothing in return. It will all work out in the end.

Until that time, be the kind of person you want to be and stand with your integrity. If it helps, get your journal, write down what you are grateful for, and say it out loud. At first, this may be difficult. Your heart may be hard at this moment. Draw on the littlest things possible to be grateful for if need be. I promise it will be worth it. Gratitude is the best weapon to fight against Satan and his evil angels that try to take over your thoughts.

You have other weapons and tools—spiritual gifts—because you are a child of God. You are of great worth. Remember, the Lord needs your help with your brothers and sisters on this earth. We are all doing the best we can. Give each other grace because that is what Jesus will do for you. Forgiving others frees you to grow. Grudges are the chains that bind us to earth and our temporal existence. Please let go. Forgive. See the eternal perspective. We are on earth like it's a big Easter egg hunt. There are opportunities all around us. The Lord wants us to help each other. Sometimes I wonder if, after death, we will see some of the hidden eggs/opportunities we missed that were hiding along our path and think, *Dang, I missed that one. That one would have been a good one to do.* I don't think we will feel a deep regret—just a missed opportunity. The quiet joy that comes from finding that egg/opportunity to help another along this earthly path.

So the question is how do we see these opportunities? If we open our hearts to the Lord, then our minds will see. The Lord loves us and wants us to have joy on earth and in the eternities. Our job is to love and help one another through the trials and experiences, the grit of life. This is only a moment in time and our time to really shape our souls. The polish will come when we return to our Heavenly Father.

That brings me to the real reason I chose to stay with my wonderful husband. In those dark moments, when I seriously considered ending the marriage, I remembered all the little miracles that brought Keith and me together in the first place. It was those little miracles that changed my mind. And here are just a few of them.

Remember the house my parents could not sell? Remember I had to find five roommates? The last roommate I found—actually, she found me—through an advertisement on the bulletin board at the Institute of

Religion for the Church of Jesus Christ of Latter-day Saints. The room was a private room and more money than she wanted to spend, but it was the only option she could find. She called me and moved in that week. I had a full house and could make the mortgage. I was relieved.

This new roommate, Kris, was from California. I loved California and the beach, so I was excited to get to know her and her experiences living there. We hung out a lot and went adventuring together. She was fun and smart and was always planning something. We had some great parties at the house. We would go dancing. She always made connections, which gave us opportunities to experience new things, and in Las Vegas, there were a great many new things to try.

She had come there to go to school, but things didn't go as planned for her. It was tough to find a job at first, and the dating scene wasn't what she expected it to be. I went with her to be her sidekick because I had a missionary I was writing to. I was waiting for him.

It was not going so well with my missionary family. There was much heartache. Kris tried to cheer me up and said I should write to her brother Keith. For a year, she told me to write to her brother. I kept telling her no. We were friends, and I didn't want to ruin a friendship or have it be weird if things didn't work out. I told her, "I don't do the brother thing."

That summer, Kris invited me to LA to see *Phantom of the Opera*. I didn't spend much money on myself in those days. I was a college student, after all, and the idea of spending $60 on myself was unheard of. I would pack a lunch or get two soft tacos for $1.29 across the street from the university to save money. I was excited to be invited but had to think about it. Deep down, I felt I must go, so I said yes.

I had never done anything like this before. We drove down in her cute white Hyundai. We got all dressed up, and the play was fabulous. That night I dreamed I married Keith. In the dream, I met his grandfather Grandpa Densley and saw the land that he lived on. I also saw secret doors at Cedar Crest that I did not know about until I actually went there. I had never seen these places or met these people. This dream is what finally pushed me to allow Keith to write to me. I told myself I would at least give it a try. It was too weird not to move forward with this impression. I was sensitive to the spirit and had had other dreams and impressions before. Kris showed me a headshot from his acting days in Hollywood, and I thought he was good looking. Kris was smart and fun to talk to, so maybe he would be too. He was attending graduate school at Humboldt State University, majoring in English. I was insecure that my letters would be red marked for improper grammar or spelling and be mailed back to me.

When Keith's first letter arrived, it was very intriguing, with his deep thoughts and fun questions. The best question was in the postscript, where he asked me, "What is your favorite fruit-colored sunset?"

He asked all his dates this and usually got a simple reply: "Orange." "Peach." Or, more creatively, "Apricot." I, being an art major, loved this question.

It so happened that a few weeks before this, I had seen an amazing sunset over the Las Vegas Valley and had to describe it to him. I responded, "Flaming red apple with plum highlights!"

That did it for him. He was intrigued, and so was I. We wrote to each other weekly and talked a couple of times a week. Long distance calls were expensive, so they were limited. We were both college students, after all. His family, who lived in Utah and California, began to visit Kris to see who I was. After his mother visited, she told Keith that he had to meet me. He scheduled his flight for September.

During our time writing letters, he sent me one photograph of him. He was standing next to his blue Mazda truck in jeans and a T-shirt with the sleeves rolled up in typical late-eighties/early nineties style. He had a full, thick head of blond hair. He looked a little like Ricky Schroder. Pictures can be deceiving, and I wondered what he would look like in person.

He was flying in on a Thursday, and for weeks, I was concerned about my missionary. *What if I like Keith? What about my missionary?*

The Monday before Keith flew into town, I got a Dear Jane letter. This is a letter from a missionary breaking up with his girlfriend. In the letter, he told me he didn't know why, but he was supposed to let me go. This letter gave me the freedom to see where things would go with Keith.

He arrived at McCarran International Airport on a Thursday, and his sister and I picked him up. When he got off the plane, and I finally got to see him in real life, my first thought was, *He's short.* He is six feet tall and not short, but I have tall brothers and have dated some taller guys, so at the moment, I thought he was short. I did think he was cute.

We had a great evening, showing off the hot downtown Las Vegas Strip. We were planning to go to Utah in the morning to visit family and see a play that other family members were a part of at Snow College, so we didn't stay out too late.

The next morning, I was afraid to come out of my room and meet him in the daylight. I thought to myself, *What if he is not as cute as he was last night? What if I was just caught up in the moment?* My nerves were racing. When I walked out of my room and greeted him in the kitchen, he was even cuter than I remembered. We spent the weekend with his family and had a great time. We continued to write and call after he got back home to Northern California.

In October, I flew to see him. He picked me up from the small airport and took me for a drive. He wanted to show me some of his favorite spots. Normally, there is fog at night, but it was a clear night with a full moon. My desert skin felt a chill with the moisture that filled the air. We went for a short walk to a point that overlooked the ocean, and on that clear night, we could see all the way to the horizon. This special place where he asked me to marry him was Wedding Rock, overlooking the Pacific coast. I said yes! I took the ring and saw three beautiful diamonds swirled in gold.

We continued our studies, and he graduated with his master's in the teaching of writing from Humboldt State University in May and moved to Las Vegas. We were married June 5, 1993, in Manti, Utah. We have three children and currently reside in Saint George, Utah.

Along our journey together, Keith and I have shared moments that felt a little like "happily ever after." There were also great regrets. Mistakes. Pain.

The world would have you believe that difficult seasons of life imply you should check out, give up, move on, do something different. Oh, it's dark and cold where you live? Fly south for the winter. Enjoy a little tropical sun. You deserve it! You can take a destination vacation, sure. Get the rest and relaxation you need. But you can't take a good vacation from life. And you're not meant to. Life's jagged edges are here to serve us. There is no escaping our destiny.

As we tumble through life, we all need a little comfort and courage. It's my prayer that in the coming months and years, you remember that you are not alone. That you once read a little book by a peculiar lady named Malissa. Maybe you laughed and cried with her as you felt her pain and realized she felt yours too.

You can probably imagine . . . this book was hard to write. But I realized in writing it how much a relatable story can mean. I'm a little (a lot?) older than you, so I've endured many more challenging experiences. May the stories that shaped me serve you too.

What's Next? We Tumble Together!

www.LifeTumbled.com

Life is best lived with other people. Other people who believe as you believe. Other people who've been where you are. Other people who want the absolute best for you. If only you knew where to find them . . .

Well, you can! Head on over to my website where you'll find a newsletter, podcast, and community of other people to tumble along life's way with. We can't wait to meet you.

www.LifeTumbled.com

About the Author

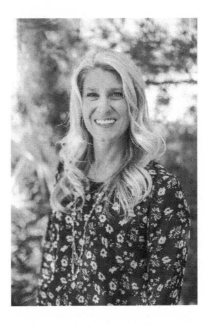

Malissa Kelsch is a wife of one, mother of three, and mother at heart of many more. As a member of the Church of Jesus Christ of Latter-day Saints, she is passionate about teaching young women entrepreneurship, industriousness, and self-sufficiency. She is building a community that supports each other as this life tumbles us around. We have one earthly life to live, so let's live it to our full potential. Connect with Malissa at www.lifetumbled.com.

Made in the USA
Columbia, SC
14 September 2021

44815156R00088